HONOR THE ANIMAL

HONOR THE ANIMAL

EXPERIENTIAL DESIGN FOR TEACHERS,
COACHES, TRAINERS, THERAPISTS,
PARENTS, AND HEALTH PROFESSIONALS

FRANK FORENCICH

ISBN (print): 978-0-9851263-6-0

Published by Frank Forencich, Bend, Oregon

HONORTHEANIMAL.EARTH

To Sebastien Alary, my best friend and inspiration for experiential design.

Also by Frank Forencich

The Enemy is Never Wrong
Activism is Medicine
Beware False Tigers
The Sapience Curriculum
Beautiful Practice

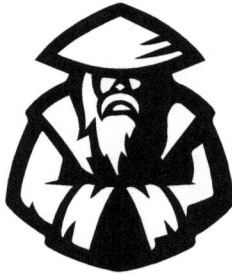

CONTENTS

The highest and most beautiful things in life are not to be heard about, nor read about, nor seen but, if one will, are to be lived.

Søren Kierkegaard

INTRODUCTION
ALL FOR ONE

Health is indivisible.

—Wendell Berry

As the song goes, "You don't know what you've got till it's gone," and for me that something was the air in my lungs, my breath, my life force, my vital energy. I was only eight years old at the time, and without warning, a vicious asthma attack brought me to my knees. My body revolted, my diaphragm convulsed, and my mind lurched into panic. And the harder I tried to regain my equanimity, the worse it got.

Fortunately, Mom was there to ease my fears. She helped me slow down, relax, and suck on the inhaler, and after a few terrifying moments, my breath returned. I was shaken but okay, for the moment at least. But in another sense, I really wasn't okay at all. My childhood was marked by a series of nagging physical afflictions. The asthma was bad enough, but I also suffered digestive troubles, allergies, and a host of skin problems. Overall, my physical vitality was tenuous, even on the good days. I tried to keep up with my friends on the athletic field, but I was always last in every event, always the weakest and the lamest. In today's language, I might well have been labeled as a case of "failure to thrive." I was a poor animal and I knew it. But Mom understood my plight and tried every remedy in sight, finally enrolling me in a swimming class, where I floundered once again. Last place in every race, I dog-paddled my way across the pool, doing my best, dominated by the healthy swimmers. But I persisted and as the months passed, my physical systems began moving in the right direction; I could almost feel the integration of organs and tissues coming together for a single purpose. I never won any races, but over the next few years, my asthma disappeared, my digestive problems abated, and by the time I graduated from high school, I was as fit and healthy as anyone in my class. To my young mind, the experience was a kind of miracle. No longer ashamed of my body and my performance, I began to feel a sense of pride and competence.

Not surprisingly, I also became fascinated with the human body and movement. In the years that followed, I journeyed the world of martial art and trained with some incredible teachers in both karate and aikido. I immersed myself in the rock climbing scene in Yosemite and discovered what my body was really capable of. As an undergraduate at Stanford, I enrolled in the program on human biology and discovered a fascinating world of evolution, neurobiology, and powerful explanations about why our bodies and behaviors are the way they are. I even traveled to Africa to learn about indigenous people and our ancestral environment.

After graduation, I continued my explorations, reading deeply about the body and the natural world, seeking out workshops and teachers across the spectrum: athletic trainers, biologists, massage therapists, physicians, and physical therapists. I even organized multi-day workshops from scratch, working with martial art team building, meditation, and presentations on health and the human predicament. Playing with my own experiential designs, I made all the usual blunders and invented a few new ones as well. But I also got a few things right.

Along the way, I began to notice something curious: Many of the teachers and professionals I listened to were talking outside their job descriptions. I heard coaches talking like therapists, teachers talking like neuroscientists, therapists talking about the role of the body in mental health, personal trainers talking like anthropologists, and physicians talking about the social and ecological determinants of health. And to top it off, a new wave of Paleo-oriented trainers was talking about the importance of human evolution and our ancestry as hunters and gatherers.

In the process, I began to see that conventional disciplinary boundaries didn't really count for much and that everyone was reaching for something bigger. In fact, everyone seemed to have a common, overlapping interest in the welfare of the human animal. I began to see an emerging confluence of attention, with everyone pointed in roughly the same direction.

This growing sense of unity has become all the more apparent with modern discoveries in the world of neuroscience and human biology. As is becoming clear, all of us—no matter our specific job descriptions—are working with the human nervous system and in particular, neuroplasticity. In fact, the primary educational and training challenge is really the same across all disciplines: creating and delivering quality experiential repetitions of the skill or capability in question. In this sense, there's little conceptual difference between teaching mathematics and coaching power lifting, between learning science and the humanities, between academic performance and performance on the athletic field. Coaches, teachers, trainers, parents, and therapists: All of us are doing essentially the same thing—nurturing the human animal with high quality life experiences.

As the years passed, I naturally began to question the entire notion of disciplinary boundaries, especially as they're applied to the human experience. As I came to see it, modern divisions between health, training, and education disciplines resemble the arbitrary geographic boundaries between nations, states, and counties. That is, the lines are gerrymandered and manipulated for convenience, not by virtue of any underlying ecological or biological foundation. In fact, the common divisions are often distracting and counterproductive; a straight line drawn across a living bioregion is just as absurd as a straight line drawn across the human body or the human experience.

Unfortunately, cultural habit dies hard. In today's marketplace, we make dozens of unnecessary distinctions between coaches and teachers, between education and training, between physical and academic education. Every specialization lays claim to its own territory, and each has its own knowledge base, journals, conferences, and best practices, but in the process, we've lost sight of the essential, unifying principles that drive human learning across all domains.

It's sometimes said that when it comes to exploring the world around us, there are only two intellectual styles:

splitters make distinctions, but lumpers seek commonalities. Splitters look for territory and are quick to enforce boundaries, while lumpers look for common themes and unifying principles. In this light, it's easy to see that modern society is dominated by splitters, specialists who claim to know everything about one increasingly narrow aspect of reality. Overwhelmed by the rising tide of information in every field, we survive by narrowing our focus, but when splitters don't talk to one another, our entire knowledge ecosystem begins to disintegrate and confusion reigns.

Going further, we might well say that modern Western culture is addicted to splitting and specialization, to knowing more and more about less and less. Some would even go so far as to say that relentless splitting is a form of violence against the natural world and in turn, a recipe for anxiety, frustration, and despair.

But the human animal has a deep psycho-spiritual craving for unity; we long for coherence. We want our bodies, our communities, and our planet to come together into some kind of integrated whole. We're quick to point fingers and weapons at other people and groups, but deep down, we really want to be one with the world and with each other.

All of which brings us around to some pivotal questions: What exactly is the work of teachers, coaches, trainers, therapists, and parents in today's world? Are we still performing our familiar roles, working the various niches that society has created for us? Or are we being drawn into something altogether different?

In a "normal," soon-to-be-bygone era, we knew our identity and our job descriptions: Coaches worked with athletes, teachers worked with students, and therapists worked with anyone who was suffering. Everyone understood their territory, their methods, and their duties.

But today, in our rapidly emerging "post-normal" era, everything will soon be up for grabs. Chaos is about to hit the fan and specializations, especially as they relate to the welfare of the human animal, are going to become increasingly fuzzy, and maybe even irrelevant. The lines will blur, pigeonholes will dissolve, and people will be forced to take on unfamiliar tasks and roles. Increasingly, teachers, coaches, trainers, and therapists will be called upon to do things they're not really trained to do.

In short, our world is about to become increasingly incoherent and challenging. Not only is our biosphere in great peril, so too is our democracy and even our humanity itself. And while turmoil is now inevitable, it's also an opportunity for a new way of working and relating to the world and to ourselves. In other words, the time has come for a true multidisciplinary flexibility. Teachers, coaches, trainers, and therapists will need a more holistic set of capabilities. It's no longer enough to camp out in isolated professional categories; now is the time to be bigger.

CHAPTER 1

PREDICAMENT

We are on the brink of an irreversible climate disaster. This is a global emergency beyond any doubt. Much of the very fabric of life on Earth is imperiled. We are stepping into a critical and unpredictable new phase of the climate crisis.

The 2024 state of the climate report: Perilous times on planet Earth

—William J Ripple, et al.
BioScience, October 2024

Before we start designing an experience for the human animal, we've got to know what we're working with. What kind of condition is the animal in? What's going on with his body, his health, his life? What does he need to thrive and function at a high level?

The need for such an assessment may well seem obvious, but then again, this is precisely the error that plagues so many conventional training and education programs. We leap into action without forethought, and we lean on existing methods and traditions while mostly ignoring the state of the creatures we're working with. But if we're going to be effective, we've got to step back and take a closer look at the animal in question and, in particular, the state of his world. If you want to know what makes the human animal tick, you've got to understand the context, the setting, and the conditions he lives in.

STATE OF THE PLANET

So we begin this exploration, as we must, with the elephant in the room: our life support system. You're surely sick of hearing the bad news by now, and you might well wonder why anyone would subject themselves to another round of grim realities. But much as we might prefer to look away, there can be no avoiding it. We have no choice but to tell the truth to ourselves and one another. To put it simply, our condition is now becoming unignorable.

What we're seeing today is a host of interconnected afflictions, a wicked cluster of wicked problems. The human animal—and the rest of life on earth—is in serious trouble. Whatever your assessment of the human predicament at this moment in history, conditions are in fact more dire than most people realize. As David Wallace-Wells put it in *The Uninhabitable Earth*, "No matter how well informed you are, you are surely not alarmed enough."

Soft language warns us about "climate change," but it's actually an "everything change." It's an ecological, social, and spiritual emergency marked by abrupt and possibly irreversible transformation of Earth systems. All the scientific fire alarms are going off. As Greta Thunberg puts it, "The house is on fire." (And the arsonists are in charge.)

Climate gets the lion's share of our attention, but this is actually a full-spectrum, three-dimensional crisis. Call it what you will: a polycrisis, a permacrisis, the Anthropocene, the Pyrocene, a mass extinction event, the Age of Consequences, or Planetary Endgame. But no matter the label, our emergency is both broad and deep. It's a public health crisis, a cultural crisis, a psychospiritual crisis, a moral crisis, a relational crisis, and a crisis of our collective imagination. All our systems are stretched to the limit: agriculture, transportation, energy, materials, medicine, education, government, human nervous systems, and in particular, the human psyche itself.

Without question, the state of the planet is the alpha crisis of our age and the most consequential challenge in human history. As author Naomi Klein has put it, "When your life support system is threatened, all other problems fit inside that problem." In other words, every other issue is secondary. When there's a gaping hole in your lifeboat, the priority is—or should be—obvious.

There's a long story here and an important history, but for our purposes, it's enough to say that our problem is one of ecological overshoot. Humanity is in the process of exceeding the biological carrying capacity of the planet, and the consequences are becoming excruciatingly obvious. Human impact in both consumption and sheer numbers is stressing every life system to the limit.

Habitat destruction and deforestation continue almost unabated, and the oceans are suffering from overheating, acidification, dead zones, and overfishing. Extreme weather is rapidly becoming a new normal, biodiversity is in steep decline, and the biomass of wild animals—in comparison to humans and human-supporting animals—is a fraction of its historical norm. According to an analysis by the World Wildlife Fund, Earth's wildlife populations have fallen, on average, by 73 percent in the past half century. Rebecca Shaw, WWF's chief scientist, described the report's findings in the bluntest possible terms: "It really does indicate to us that the fabric of nature is unraveling."

According to Planetary Boundaries Science, an international scientific partnership established in 2023 in affiliation with Planetary Guardians, six of Earth's nine planetary boundaries have already been breached: climate change, biosphere integrity, land system change, freshwater change, biogeochemical flows, and the introduction of novel chemical and genetic entities. If the planet was a human body, this would be a genuine medical emergency.

Sadly, casual observers fail to understand the nature of complex Earth system dynamics and, in turn, the urgency of the situation. Most of us are inclined to think about the world in linear terms, with small, incremental change that takes place over long periods of time, and in this light, future disruptions seem trivial.

But the biosphere and atmosphere are immensely complex, highly dynamic systems that behave in distinctly nonlinear ways. Change takes place, then feeds on itself in positive feedback loops that amplify and accelerate the process. If left unchecked and unregulated, these systems cross tipping points and enter into entirely new domains of function. When this happens, there's no going back to the original condition; the change is irreversible. This is what keeps earth scientists up at night. If we continue on this course, large portions of our Earth may well become uninhabitable, much sooner than we expect. In other words, tomorrow is *not* going to be like today.

STATE OF THE ANIMAL

The state of the planet is horrifying enough, but what about the state of *us*? How is the human animal faring under these drastically unprecedented conditions? To answer these questions, we might be inclined to seek out physicians and health experts, but sadly, our modern medicalized orientation is often myopic and narrowly focused on the state of individuals.

For example, we say that patients have a neurotransmitter deficiency or a "noncommunicable lifestyle disease." We run tests and order diagnostic imaging, narrowing our field of vision to the condition of particular tissues and organs. If that fails to provide an explanation, we narrow our search once again, looking to the individual's DNA and genes to tell us what we want to know. But this is big-picture blindness, a failure to appreciate context and setting. In the words of the statesman Václav Havel, modern medicine—especially in the domain of mental health—is dominated by "those who do not look outside airplane windows."

But humans are hypersocial animals living in an ecological context. The world outside our skin is constantly impacting our health and function, turning genes on and off, influencing the flow of informational substances, altering our microbiome, giving us our sense of safety or danger and altering the activity of our autonomic nervous systems. In other words, the natural and social world literally sculpts our bodies, our cognition, our health, and in turn, our behavior.

When we view the human animal in isolation, we see ourselves *in vitro*, literally meaning "within glass." But our most vital work is to see the animal in context, or as biologists put it, *in vivo*. So let's suppose that you're a veterinarian from Mars. You've traveled to Earth and parked your spaceship in low-Earth orbit, where you can get a good view of the creatures and ecosystems below. You've got a particular interest in the species *Homo sapiens*, and you're wondering how that animal is getting along. How is this creature faring? Is it thriving or suffering? What are you to make of the modern human condition and the state of the human animal on Earth?

In short, things are not looking good. In the world of conservation biology and environmental activism, writers often quote a passage from Aldo Leopold's *Sand County Almanac*: "One of the penalties of an ecological education is that one lives alone in a world of wounds." It's an apt description of our ecological predicament, but the same might well be said of the human animal. To paraphrase Leopold, we might say that one of the penalties of a public health education is that we become increasingly aware of human suffering; we too live "in a world of wounds."

Once we understand how the human animal works, it becomes very hard to unsee the traumas, stresses, and other afflictions that compromise our well-being. The list is long and painful to read, but if we're going to be effective experiential designers for the human animal, a review is essential:

MISMATCH

Our problems begin with the contrast between our ancestral bodies and today's modern environment. Sometimes described as the "evolutionary discordance hypothesis," it's easier to simply call it mismatch. In short, we've evolved to survive in a very different world than the one we inhabit today.

To get an idea of how stark the difference is, just consider the contrasts and alien qualities of the modern world. Today we live in an alien:

physical environment, in which buildings, vehicles, and chairs force us into sedentary and chronically flexed postures.

circadian environment, in which artificial light profoundly disrupts our sleep-wake cycle.

nutritional environment, in which food—even when real—is geographically isolated from its natural source.

social environment, with ambiguous and often confusing relationships and rules about appropriate behavior.

sensory environment, dominated by noise and hypernormal sensations.

material environment, our tissues constantly under assault by a witch's brew of endocrine disruptors, air pollution, pesticides, fertilizers, microplastics, and novel substances that have never existed in nature.

microbial environment, the microbiome inside and outside our bodies drastically modified by the overuse of antiseptics, antibiotics, pesticides, and herbicides.

mental and spiritual environment, dominated by synthetic for-profit narratives that have little or nothing to do with actual human needs.

moral environment, in which ends now dominate over means, where calculation, self-interest, and ulterior motives take priority over our universal humanity.

Taken together, these alien qualities challenge us to the core. It's bad enough that modern conditions are so often unfamiliar to our ancestral bodies, but they also force us into behaviors that are drastically out of step with our evolutionary origins. In short, our alien environment sculpts our nervous systems into some absolutely abnormal patterns of living and being. Some people do manage to live and even thrive under these conditions, but for many others, it all comes down to a slow-motion trauma that grinds away at our bodies and spirits.

DOMESTICATION

Closely related to mismatch is our transformation from wild human animals to domesticated, often passive actors who are unaware of their innate powers and strength. Beginning with agriculture and settlement, we abandoned our nomadic, hunting-and-gathering ways and began to suffer a gradual loss of freedom to move our bodies through the world; we lost our *vagility*.

Drawn from the world of wildlife ecology, this word refers to a creature's ability to move through habitat without constraint. Every species has its own requirements and preferred range, but we now know that restricting a creature's vagility has severe consequences for its health, brain function, and psychology. Animals in captivity struggle with this constantly.

But today, the vagility of the human animal is massively compromised by urbanization and the built environment. Most of us like to think we have freedom, but in a wickedly overcrowded world, it's actually a rare luxury. Affluent people can move with less restriction, but for everyone else, modern living often feels like a kind of incarceration.

We begin to feel less like animals and more like cogs in a vast, oppressive machine.

RELATIONAL DYSFUNCTION

Mismatch and domestication are bad enough, but we're also confronted by a wickedly unfamiliar social world. Almost everyone is aware of the bitter partisanship, polarization, and division that characterize modern society, but we're also suffering from an erosion of trust that compromises everything we're trying to do. Deception seems to be everywhere now: Marketing and advertising firms stretch the truth to the breaking point, politicians traffic in exaggerated, even fabricated claims, and the Internet amplifies every fear a thousand-fold.

So it's no wonder that we're seeing a distressing xenophobic survival strategy for modern life: Don't pick up the phone unless you recognize the number, don't click on a link unless you absolutely have to, and don't believe a word anyone outside your circle tells you. Cons are everywhere—so we believe—so the safest course is to keep your head down and ignore the rest.

At the same time, we're massively distressed by the abnormal, isolating quality of modern relationships. The frenetic pace of commerce forces us into increasingly frequent transactional encounters—what we might call "short relationships." In a typical day, we might see and talk to many people, but much of this contact is confined to the buying, selling, or delivery of products and services; beyond the legal and procedural details, there's not much humanity involved. In this kind of sterilized environment, it's no surprise to see a breakdown of community and an epidemic of loneliness.

This is the paradox of life on an overstressed, hyperactive planet; it's becoming increasingly difficult to find people with the time for a relaxed, meaningful human interaction. In other words, there's no time for authentic human rapport. Everything's rushed, scripted, managed, monetized, and calculated for maximum financial return. To put it another way, what we're experiencing might well be called "relational deprivation" and a "hardening of the self." As a culture, we've gone all in on the welfare and happiness of the isolated individual; marketing messages are all about me and you, but rarely about *us*. In fact, an entire lexicon has grown up around the human animal as an isolated, stand-alone entity. Every day we hear about the importance of self-awareness, self-acceptance, self-confidence, self-esteem, self-optimization, self-realization, self-actualization, self-mastery, self-control, self-love, self-care, self-worth, self-improvement, and self-sufficiency. It's no wonder that New York Times columnist David Brooks calls this culture "The Big Me."

ALIENATION

At the same time, our relationship with nature has become increasingly tenuous, distant, and distorted. As our lives become increasingly urbanized, it takes more and more effort to get to the Big Outside, and with so many indoor seductions, many of us simply opt to stay home. But modern buildings are intentionally engineered to keep us insulated from heat, cold, moisture, and nature at large. In turn, we no longer feel the qualities, textures, sounds, and sensations of the living world.

It's a problem of both deficit and excess, of *hypo* and *hyper*, of too little and too much. Our sensory experience is hypo in the sense that modern people can go days, weeks, even months touching only smooth, inert, plasticized objects and surfaces: our keyboards and trackpads, our phones, our granite counter-tops, and our faux leather steering wheels. And if we live in a "low touch" social circle, we might go long periods without ever touching another human body.

At the same time, we're inundated by a flood of hypernormal sensations: nearly constant noise, artificially flavorful food products engineered for maximum craving and desire, amplified music piped directly into our ear canals, unnatural colors on the screens of our devices, and now, artificially generated images of people, places, and events that would never occur in a historically normal, natural environment.

It's no wonder that we're on edge. When our sensory experience is radically altered, there are bound to be consequences that extend beyond the sensations themselves. In fact, the mental and spiritual health of the human animal depends in large measure on what we might call the "touch-brain connection." We need natural sensation to keep us grounded in reality, to feel a continuity with the living earth. When that sensation is absent or distorted, our connection with life itself becomes sketchy, unreliable, and unsatisfying.

ACCELERATION

Our psycho-physical distress is compounded by the ferocious, accelerating, and generally senseless pace of modern living. For the vast majority of human experience on this planet, living conditions didn't change much and people were never in any great hurry to do anything. Apart from local, mostly subtle changes to plants, animals, seasons, and weather, human life would have been generally stable from year to year and from generation to generation. This relaxed pace of living persisted across hundreds of generations, but in a veritable instant, human life picked up speed and has been accelerating ever since.

Beginning with the scientific and industrial revolution, amplified by the printing press, new technologies brought an avalanche of novelty to the human experience, a rate of change for which our bodies and minds were completely unprepared. We struggle to catch up, but our predicament is compounded by an unconscious stress response. Uncomfortable in our predicament, our impulse is to simply go faster, lurching into the future, not with a particular sense of purpose, but as an escape from ambiguity. Unable to sit still, we drive ourselves into a frenzy, a condition the Japanese call "the hurry disease."

Not surprisingly, our ability to concentrate is also diminishing. Faced with an onslaught of complexity, novelty, and acceleration, our attention is fragmenting; we're bringing less and less of our creative attention to bear on a world that's becoming more challenging by the minute. But the human mind can only tolerate so much chaos-tasking; with every shift of attention, we burn up our precious cognitive and psychological resources.

STRESS

The acceleration and complexification of the modern world drives our angst and imposes an almost unbearable stress burden on the human animal. Fire hosed with ambiguous information and vague threats, we feel ourselves losing control. Fear and urgency are in the air now, surging through our collective unconscious. Especially in the digital world, our lives feel precarious; all it takes is one misplaced swipe or click to ruin your financial or social life—or so it seems.

The consequence is that a significant number—even a majority—of modern people are now living in survival mode, ever alert to modern versions of lions, tigers, and bears. To put it in neurological terms, a large number of us are living with a hypersensitized amygdala (the warning center of the brain), weakened hippocampus (memory center), and weakened prefrontal cortex (impulse control and executive function).

This adds up to some particularly dangerous large-scale consequences that affect our entire culture. The problem is that stress doesn't just compromise our individual health, it also degrades our cognition and behavior. When we're chronically stressed, we become hypervigilant, suspicious, and xenophobic. In turn, this manifests as polarization and toxic tribalism (tribe over truth). Our creativity contracts and, in the process, we become increasingly neophobic (fear of new ideas and experiences). Likewise, our stress drives a powerful but largely unconscious reversion to the familiar: we retreat to familiar experiences, people, and ideas, no matter their inherent quality or value.

To make matters worse, we contract into self-interest and start hoarding power, money, tools, and possessions as a hedge against an ambiguous future. We become obsessed with safety and short-term perspectives, and when things get really threatening, we fall back on reflexive obedience, conformity, and in the creative arts, cliché. In short, stress cripples our equanimity and our creativity, just at the moment when we need it the most.

EXISTENTIAL VACUUM

Naturally, our predicament is also reflected in a distortion of our values. In the modern world, nothing's sacred, not even our life-supporting systems. We dishonor our nature as animals, our physicality, our history, and our ancestry. Chronically overworked, undersupported, and overstressed, our bodies have been reduced to little more than a labor source for the capitalist enterprise. For many of us, productivity is the only game in town.

In fact, the way we treat our bodies and our humanity is a simple reflection of the way we treat our habitat and the world at large: as a resource to be mined and exploited, as a means to a profitable end. Just as we strip mine the land for minerals and the ocean for protein, so too do we squeeze the human animal for anything we can monetize. In the process, we diminish and disrespect our animal nature. In our frenetic rush to progress, we're literally leaving ourselves behind.

Even our vision is contracting. Overwhelmed with stress and uncertainty, we fail to see the interdependence of life on Earth and we're even becoming blind to our ultimate reliance on natural systems. In our failure to honor our ancestry and our physicality, we've forgotten our relational nature, our sense of meaning, and our innate powers. Legendary psychologist Viktor Frankl described this condition as an "existential vacuum." We're adrift, lost in a psychic wilderness of our own creation.

LIFE IN THE QUAGMIRE

All of which puts the human animal into a wicked mental health quagmire of addiction, depression, anxiety, and related neurological afflictions. People are suffering, not because of flaws in their personal brain chemistry but rather because of the conditions in which they live. Modern medicine mistakenly places the origin of mental illness squarely on the shoulders of the individual sufferer, but the pandemic of mental anguish cannot be understood as an affliction that just happens to large numbers of isolated individuals. Rather, it's about the nature of the modern system itself.

To be sure, some people do manage to adapt and find ways to flourish in the midst of alien, stressful, and dehumanizing conditions, and sometimes the human animal does prevail in the face of body-hostile processes and forces. But the odds are long and, even worse, all of these social and environmental pressures are likely to become even more pronounced in the near future. As bioregions and habitat break down and resources become depleted, the effect on the human animal will become extreme.

As physician Gabor Maté has shown—especially in books such as *The Myth of Normal*—trauma is far more widespread than most of us recognize. The modern world, for all its comforts and conveniences, can be an incoherent, alienating, and unfriendly place. If you manage to run the gauntlet of education, relationships, housing, money, and career, you can live a satisfying and body-friendly life. But for those who miss a step along the way, the consequences can be severe. Modern society can be brutally unkind to those who miss a beat.

In fact, repeated frustration leads the human animal—any animal in fact—to assume helplessness and powerlessness in general. In turn, this leads to weakness and capitulation, all of which feeds on itself in a cycle of resignation and hopelessness. In essence, we're experiencing a planet-wide epidemic of learned helplessness, and even worse, the condition is wickedly contagious. As hypersocial animals, we pay close attention to one another's sense of optimism or pessimism, and people's general attitude in the face of adversity. Just as individuals can come to assume failure, so too can entire social groups. And when groups become helpless, this becomes fertile ground for autocrats, tyrants, and corporate opportunists (disaster capitalists) to step in and seize control.

Any of these mental health challenges, if imposed on the human animal overnight, would become instantly apparent, and presumably, we would act in our own defense. If an alien power came to Earth and imposed these conditions upon us, we would presumably have fought back. But like frogs in a pan of slowly warming water, we adapt and adjust, even as our peril grows. The human animal is in big trouble, but the party goes on.

NO IS NOT ENOUGH

Overwhelmed with bad news, complexity, and ambiguity, many of us fall into despair and some days we can scarcely bring ourselves to face the grim realities of ecocide, political dysfunction, cultural gridlock, and declining public health. It all feels like an uphill fight now, our personal Davids facing an army of powerful, ruthless, and heavily financed Goliaths.

We do what we can with our personal efforts, but it all feels insignificant or even futile. We try to stay as healthy as possible. We cut back or eliminate air travel, cut back or eliminate meat consumption, scaling back our impact to a graceful and meaningful life-supporting minimum.

At the same time, we do what we can to resist the rising tide of ecocide and fascism. We may not have much in the way of political, economic, or cultural power, but we're not going quiet into the dark night either.

This *no* of resistance and revolution is vital and honorable. Healthy human animals are right to push back against forces and agents that would destroy their life-support systems and their health. We're right to set boundaries by saying *no* to habitat destruction, imperialism, racism, and injustice. But as author Naomi Klein has put it, "No is not enough." Rebellion is a first step on the path to transformation, but there also needs to be a creation, a building—an art project, if you will. To put it another way, our *no* is necessary but is not sufficient. To have a shot at a functional future, there must also be an intentional, ferociously creative *yes*.

In this spirit, now would be an excellent time to double down on the human body and to nurture our primal human capabilities, the innate powers that have sustained us for hundreds of thousands of years. To put it another way, our primary objective is to bring the human animal back to life. In this effort, we prioritize not just biomedical health and the absence of disease but the entire experience of being vibrant, competent, and resourceful beings. In other words, we need an antidote to our amnesia. We need to re-inhabit our bodies and remember who we are: powerful, adaptable, creative, and intelligent animals. To put it simply, we need experiences that help people become outrageously, radically human.

Reflecting on the scourge of world war in the early twentieth century, the historian and writer H.G. Wells once warned that "civilization is in a race between education and catastrophe." It was true in his day and even more so today, but this is much more than a call for improved academic education. Rather, it's a call for something deeper and more elemental. If Wells were alive today, he might well say that we're in a race between creativity and catastrophe, between functional human beings and the socioecological collapse of our life-support systems. In other words, the fate of our world literally hinges on the health, capability, and imagination of the human animal.

Naturally, critics will push back on this suggestion and protest that prioritizing the human animal would be unduly expensive and inconvenient; taking care of people simply costs too much. But the thing to remember is that what we have *now* is massively expensive, inconvenient, counterproductive, and harmful to both humans and nonhuman life. Unsupported, chronically stressed, and traumatized people don't just suffer personal pain and mental illness, they also fail to make the kind of creative contributions we so desperately need. In the long run, prioritizing the human animal would actually be the most productive and least expensive thing we could do.

EXPERIENCE IS THE LANGUAGE OF THE BODY

> A man who carries a cat by the tail learns a lesson he can learn in no other way.
>
> —Mark Twain

This is where experiential design comes into play. As teachers, coaches, parents, trainers, and therapists, we all want the best for the human animal, and we'd like to shape our programs and curriculums to meet that need. Unfortunately, many of us are constrained by tradition; the experiences we currently deliver to our patients, children, and students are often handed to us by institutions and organizations, much of it in the form of templates and boilerplate.

As individuals, we have the best of intentions, but in many settings, we're delivering experiences that haven't been crafted with the human animal in mind. Our elders were trying their best, but they didn't really know much about neurobiology, the autonomic nervous system, the social determinants of health, or the nature of stress. If they had, our schools, gyms, homes, and workplaces would look entirely different than they do today.

Experiential design may sound like a fancy new thing, and in some ways it is, but many of us already have some familiarity with the design process and we see glimpses of the practice in many domains: Wedding planners pay close attention to detail, restaurant owners and chefs craft menus, yoga teachers plan retreats, interior designers create indoor spaces, architects and urban planners work with built environments, and so on, all of it with an eye toward creating the best possible experiences for clients and customers. So yes, while many of us have some familiarity with the practice of experiential design, what we lack is a big vision, an expansive view of the human animal in the world.

With this in mind, our experiential design process will take a radically upstream, "start from scratch" orientation that questions everything about training, coaching, therapy, and education. We might even call it a veterinary approach to training and caring for people. The objective is simple: honor and develop the adaptive, creative, and pro-future capabilities of the human animal.

The good news is that neuroscience has a great deal to teach us about the power of experience in shaping our bodies and our minds. A solid body of research has overturned the grim dogma of a static nervous system—*neurofatalism*—and replaced it with a far more promising understanding of plasticity and *neuro-optimism*.

In short, we now know that the nervous system is highly dynamic and is constantly remodeling itself according to how it's used. Microscopic changes to the nervous system are all, in the language of the field, "use dependent." In other words, experience is the primary—even the exclusive—driver of plasticity. Or, to put it another way, experience is the original, implicit language of the body. We learn precisely what we live; no more and no less.

When we think about it, we begin to realize that it could hardly be any other way. When we're born, life takes us by surprise. Suddenly and inexplicably, we appear in the world vulnerable, incompetent, and completely at the mercy of the conditions around us. No one prepared us for this. Mom's experience shaped our tissue in utero, and her body prepared us for the conditions that *she* was living in but ultimately, it was just us and the world. It was our experience—either nurturing or stressful—that told our bodies how to develop.

As we grew into adulthood, our experiences continued to exert a powerful influence on our bodies, our thinking, and our behavior. Those encounters may have been nurturing and rhythmically predictable, or incoherent, confusing, and hostile. But no matter the details, it was experience that sculpted our bodies, our nervous systems, our brains, our expectations, and ultimately, our relationships with the world at large. It was our experience—not cognition or verbal instruction—that made us who we are.

Perhaps this seems self-evident, maybe even trivial. But how then to explain the fact that modern educational and training practices largely ignore this bedrock principle? After all, the modern educational landscape is littered with hundreds of narrow techniques, programs, modalities, technologies, and methods, most of which are dominated by cognitive, top-down, Cartesian assumptions. If we can just get people to sit still long enough, we can pump their brains full of the required information, test their understanding, and then move on. But none of this is grounded in neuroscience or evolutionary biology, and it's no surprise that it so often leaves us mired in frustration.

To put it bluntly, today's approach to the human animal constitutes what some might call an "epic fail" of creative intelligence. In other words, our modern priorities are wildly out of proportion. We go to incredible lengths to design every detail of our cars, our websites, our computers, and other physical products, but when it comes to training, educating, and taking care of people, we rarely stop to wonder how design thinking might apply. Even more to the point, we don't even seem to think that such experiences can or should be designed at all. We simply take what's handed to us, rearrange the deck chairs, and hope for the best.

This is no longer acceptable. The time has come for intentional, deliberate design for training, educating, and healing ourselves. Above all, we need to honor experience as the master influencer, the master trainer, and the master coach for the human animal. We like to think that our words and ideas are moving people, and sometimes they do, but in the end, experience is the ultimate teacher for most of us, most of the time. In the long run, experience is what sticks.

HONOR THE ANIMAL

As someone who works with the human animal, you've probably wondered a good deal about all of this. You're curious about creating transformational experiences for your students, clients, patients, offspring, or athletes, and you'd like to inspire people to new levels of performance, integration, and meaning. This book is about making just this kind of magic. It's about creating culture and programs that get people moving and working together in ways that are consistent with their ancestry and are relevant to the world we're living in.

The potential here is immense. When we get people together and prime them with the right kinds of engagement, their bodies respond with intelligence and equanimity. They discover a sense of physicality and social rapport that might well be missing in their daily lives. You'll see it in their eyes, their faces, their voices, and their postures. When we honor their animal nature, people respond with vitality and exuberance. This is why we do it.

As you'll see, there are any number of ways to use the material in this book. You can put these ideas to work in schools, gyms, clinics, studios, or living rooms. Or maybe you're a dabbler and you'd like to cherry-pick some ideas for your personal use. Maybe you'll only put a fraction of this material to work in your life, or maybe you're more ambitious and want to go all in on experiential design. Maybe you'd like to create your own workshops or retreats and bring in people from all over the world.

Or, maybe you're not a professional at all. Maybe you're a parent who's trying to take care of your children and make sure that their lives are off to a good start. Naturally, you'll be taking on a variety of roles along the way; sometimes you'll be a teacher, a coach, a trainer, or a therapist, or maybe just a friend. And while it's fun to joke about children who behave "like animals," it's also perfectly accurate. No matter our age, we're all *Homo sapiens*, with the same basic biology, psychology, and needs. Age differences are real and should be honored, but in the end, we all live and learn by the same principles. By understanding the power of experience in human development and behavior, you can make a real difference in the lives of the people that you serve.

In any case, this book is designed to clear your mind and get you thinking in new ways about education, training, coaching, and teaching. But bear in mind that some of the solutions offered here are intentionally utopian. That is, we start by thinking big and ignoring practical limitations about what's possible. In this effort, a panoramic view is essential. A massively disruptive storm is upon us and we're living on the cusp of radical social and ecological change. Convention is breaking apart and new opportunities will soon arise. Like it or not, you'll be forced to improvise and create, maybe on the fly, and maybe without support. As our current paradigm collapses, you might well be left with a handful of semi-functional fragments and no idea what to do next.

So forget the practicalities, at least for the moment. Forget the fact that your organization doesn't have the resources, the time, or the money to make any of this happen. Forget the fact that tradition and bureaucracies are stacked against you. Orient your thinking toward the needs of the human animal, then look for opportunities as they arise.

You can also think of this book as an antidote to the despair that often comes with work in health and education professions. Living in this time of chaos, bad news, and frequent defeats, many of us—most of us, perhaps— are inclined to hopelessness. But focused action is a solution in itself, independent of any outward success or victory. This is the power of *ikigai*, the Japanese concept of meaning and purpose: As soon as we begin moving with intention and a sense of direction, the body-mind begins to integrate around a single objective. Working with experiential design can give you just such a purpose.

Naturally, you'll be challenged along the way. Your creative efforts at experiential design will strike some people as unorthodox, even unacceptable. You'll be violating conventional boundaries and people will push back. Governing bodies, insurance companies, and colleagues will tell you to stay in your lane and stick to the approved script, whatever that might be.

All of which might dampen your enthusiasm, but don't be alarmed. In fact, your scope of practice is actually much broader than institutional rules would suggest. Your beat is the human body, the human animal, and the human future, so stick with it. You'll be doing good work and moving in the right direction. Taking care of the human animal is a noble and honorable practice. If other people want to stay mired in archaic, outdated methods and orientations, that's up to them. You've got more important things to do.

CHAPTER 2
STARTING FROM SCRATCH

In the beginner's mind there are many possibilities, but in the expert's, there are few.

—Shunryu Suzuki
Zen Mind, Beginner's Mind: Informal Talks on Zen Meditation and Practice

Empty your cup, Grasshopper. Now is the time to clear away your preconceptions and conditioning about how people learn, grow, and heal. To put it another way, let's begin our exploration with some intentional amnesia. Forget everything you know, or think you know, about how education, coaching, parenting, and training ought to be conducted. Forget about standard curriculums, grade levels, performance standards, best practices, periodization, drills, exercises, and convention. Forget about your favorite discipline, your favorite sport, and your favorite training practices. Forget your elders, your professors, your colleagues, and your textbooks. Wipe your mind clean and start with fresh eyes.

Now, let's suppose that you're tasked with creating some

kind of optimal training and learning experiences for the modern human animal, completely from scratch. What would such programs look and feel like? How would you organize them? What kind of drills, games, and presentations would you include? What would be the tone and purpose of your effort? As we've seen, the human animal is in serious trouble, so what would be the vital elements in your design?

As an individual, you might be new to this game and you might well feel that it's a heavy lift to answer these questions on your own. So let's imagine a team approach. Suppose you had the resources to assemble a team of physicians, teachers, trainers, therapists, coaches, and public health experts. Add in some veterinarians, evolutionary biologists, trauma specialists, zoologists, animal behavior specialists, neuroscientists, and interpersonal neurobiologists. Then, just to round things out, add some artists, musicians, drummers, and dancers to the mix.

This would be a true multidisciplinary team, dedicated to designing optimal, radically human learning and training experiences. But what would their creation look and feel like? What would their objectives be? The human animals of planet Earth are obviously struggling to create a functional future, so what kind of training and educational experience would your team create? Confronted by a population of humans in various states of health, education, and performance, what would be your experiential prescription?

OBJECTIVES

It's a massive undertaking, but we can narrow it down by focusing on our goals. What do we hope to accomplish with our experiential designs? What do we want for the human animals that we work with? Naturally, there will be plenty of discussion and outright dissent on the matter, but the first point is often lost in the process.

That is, no matter the domain, objectives are vital to success. There's got to be some kind of consensus as to what we're trying to do, and that consensus should be clear and repeated often to everyone involved. There should never be any doubt about where we're going or why we're doing what we're doing.

But sadly, this is where we often fail. As trainers, coaches, parents, and educators, we plunge into our various practices, excited to get to the important stuff, but without a clear understanding of where we're going. We send our students and clients into action with vague notions of wellness, success, happiness, fitness, performance, or academic excellence, but with little attention to our existential predicament.

So, in keeping with our big-picture thinking on experiential design, let's consider a truly ambitious goal. Given the nature of our planetary predicament, the tenuous condition of the human animal, and the outlook for increasing chaos and stress around the world, there's a compelling need to maintain our humanity, creativity, and equipoise in the face of adversity and dehumanizing forces. To put it another way, we need to nurture high-functioning people, people who can show up in the midst of extremely difficult circumstances and remain creative. We're looking for people who can maintain their equanimity and equipoise, even in the face of social stress and ecological chaos.

This sounds like a good start, but what exactly is a high-functioning human, anyway? In popular conversation, we're quick to recognize and complain about dysfunctional people who can't hold a job, sustain a conversation, or fulfill the demands of daily life. But how do we identify a high-functioning person? What kind of qualities would she have? How would high-functioning people behave in the face of stress, ambiguity, and uncertainty? You're free to draw up your own description, but in the meantime, here are some ideas to get you started:

Alive. It's a tragedy that we even need to say this but, above all, the high-functioning human is alive, which is to say, she's a vigorous, physical being. Her body is vibrant and she's actively engaged in the experience of daily living. She identifies with her physicality. Strong and endurant, she enjoys bringing her body to bear in every moment. She likes being powerful and is able to withstand common physical stressors. Far more than conventional fitness, this is a deep orientation toward our primal, animal heritage.

Awake. Not only is the high-functioning human physically engaged, she's also alert and attentive to the world. She's vulnerable to experience, which is to say, she's willing to look reality in the face and revise her beliefs and behavior as necessary. She's intensely curious and refuses to fall for the consumerist lullaby or synthetic narratives. To put it another way, she's left Plato's cave, the chamber of comfortable illusion that keeps us isolated from real life on the outside.

Adapted and adaptable. In her relationship to the world, our high-functioning human is both adapted *and* adaptable. She's fluent and capable with current conditions but flexible enough to create new behaviors in new circumstances. When forced into unusual or unfamiliar settings, she observes keenly and develops new skills on the fly. She holds her habits lightly and is willing to try new ways of living. In essence, the high-functioning human is a life-long learner.

Liberally educated. To put it another way, our high-functioning human is liberally educated, which is to say, she has an expanded sense of space and time, including a sense of history and the wider world of human experience. Both a specialist and a generalist, she strives to know something about everything and everything about something. Fluent in both science and the humanities, she's capable of navigating diverse challenges and novel experiences.

Grounded. Our high-functioning human is also grounded, which is to say, she's realistic in her understanding and assessment of conditions. Living in an ambiguous and sometimes chaotic world, she knows the difference between what's truly dangerous and what's merely distracting. In other words, she's capable of distinguishing between real tigers and false tigers. She isn't easily seduced by superficial anxieties but keeps her eye on genuine risks, both to herself and those around her. This gives her the ability to stay balanced and equipoised, even when challenged by stressful events.

Creative and adventurous. As an aspiring artist, the high-functioning human is naturally creative, curious, and adventurous. She wonders what's out there and is never quite satisfied with the status quo. She wants to know about the nature of the world and her capacity for learning. She has an active, practical imagination that shows her new ways to interact and live. She's willing to take creative risks to make something new.

Socially fluent. Living in community, the high-functioning human is socially competent, with the ability to navigate diverse, sometimes ambiguous social situations. Sensitive to others, she can converse and interact with a wide range of people. She appreciates the human universals that animate people around the world and is quick to find common interests and values. She cares about other people and their sufferings.

Skillful. The high-functioning human is practically skillful and handy with daily challenges. She's mastered basic skills with hand tools, simple machines, digital devices, and common materials. She has the ability to make repairs, fixes, and workarounds for practical problems. In the face of difficult circumstances, these skills give her a sense of competence, mastery, and confidence.

Engaged. Finally, the high-functioning human is an engaged, active participant in the world. To put it another way, she holds an activist orientation. Never apathetic or escapist, she takes responsibility for conditions as they exist. She's prepared to stand up, speak out, and assume leadership in high-stress conditions.

She feels fear like any other human animal, but she also possesses a sense of physical, moral, and social courage—a willingness to accept risk in pursuit of a better world.

PRESCRIPTION

Obviously, this description of our idealized, high-functioning human animal sets a high bar and we might well wonder if anyone can truly be and do all these things. Nevertheless, it's important to have an aspiration that will help us shape and execute our designs. When faced with decisions and dilemmas as to how our training and coaching should unfold, we can always refer back to our objective. Does the exercise, drill, game, or experience in question contribute to the development of high-functioning humans? If not, we might want to try another approach.

In turn, this brings us to yet another set of questions. What kind of program, event, or experience would we like to create? What if we had the resources, time and social support we needed to create something truly original? Suppose you had the opportunity to tweak established traditions to make something more humane and effective; what would such an experience look and feel like? Returning to our original thought experiment, what kind of experiential prescription would our space-faring veterinarians offer for the human animals on Earth?

A holistic model. Without question, our interdisciplinary team would almost certainly begin with the notion that our programs and experiences should be as holistic and integrating as possible. In the popular imagination, we're quick to think of the common formulation of mind-body-spirit, but that's only one possibility. In 1977, physician George Engel proposed a more expansive theory of illness and healing that he called the *biopsychosocial* model, integrating body, mind, and society. Likewise, native and indigenous people have long held a six-part model that includes mind-body-spirit-land-tribe-ancestry. Or, we might look to this model described by three concentric circles of life support: habitat, tribe and community, and meaning.

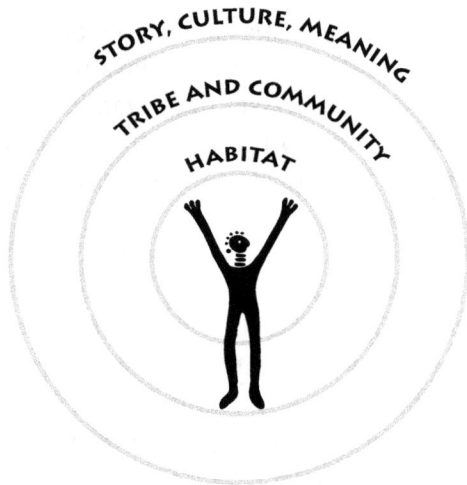

All of these models are useful, but they're also intimidating in their scope. It's hard enough to coach or teach any one skill or aptitude, much less have the time, expertise, and resources to make our programs truly comprehensive. In theory, it could take years or even decades to offer a truly well-rounded experience to our students, patients, and athletes, and practically speaking, decisions and choices must be made. Nevertheless, we can and should strive for the holistic ideal; even when specializing, our focus should always be on the whole human animal.

An upstream approach. With this in mind, our interdisciplinary team would begin by prescribing experiences that honor beginnings. That is, we'd look for a *salutogenic* (health + origins) orientation that goes to the source of human health and learning. The closer we can get to the psychological, neurological, and social points of origin, the more effective we can be. Downstream solutions are sometimes necessary, but the real power lies in the first moments. As Shakespeare put it, "Meet the first beginnings. Look to the budding mischief before it has time to ripen to maturity."

An interconnected view. Next, our experiences would honor life itself, especially the three-billion-year celebration of biological exuberance that we see in the natural world. Think of E. O. Wilson's biophilia, our "innate tendency to affiliate with life and life-like processes." This is an ancient, biocentric view of the world, an orientation in which humans see themselves not as masters but as participants in the flux and flow of life. This perspective offers a vital antidote to our culture of human exceptionalism and the sense of separation, anxiety, and disconnection that comes with it.

A truthful voice. Likewise, we'd recognize and honor the depth, scope, and extremity of the modern human predicament. In our teaching and coaching, there would be no attempt to minimize or sugarcoat the gravity of our situation; we'd tell the truth about all of it. We'd be upfront about the challenges we face and we'd promote a life of relevance. Both explicitly and implicitly, our programs would help people understand and act in the world as it exists.

A physical practice. Naturally, our experiences would honor and prioritize the needs of the human body, the ultimate source of our vitality, our sensitivity, and our intelligence. Our experience would be genuinely physical, with vigorous engagement and participation. Exertion and participation are the essential elements in building our vitality and capability; we'd provide direct encounters with people, habitat, and the task at hand.

Throughout the process, we'd respect human ancestry, both biological and indigenous. Humans have a rich history that informs everything that we do, think, and believe; every aspect of our anatomy, physiology, and psychology is the way it is because of our history in wild, outdoor settings. Without a sense of origins, we're adrift.

A communal outlook. Naturally, we'd honor and respect our hypersocial nature, especially the findings and implications of social neuroscience and interpersonal neurobiology. Everyone knows that hypersocial humans learn best in groups. We like to face a shared predicament together, with a unifying narrative about what we're trying to do. Likewise, we'd honor the human universals that animate all human beings, regardless of their origins or culture. Wonder, language, play, music, craft, connection, social relationship, and hope for a better future are common to all people, everywhere.

A compassionate orientation. Finally, we'd acknowledge the reality of human stress, trauma, and suffering.

Humans are laboring under a heavy stress burden, and our experiences would offer a supportive, humanizing antidote. We'd honor individual differences, listening, and sharing. We'd demonstrate equity, inclusiveness, safe expression, safe touch, and compassion. In Bessel van der Kolk's prescription, we'd provide experiences that "deeply and viscerally contradict the helplessness, rage or collapse that result from trauma."

Obviously, this idealized prescription amounts to yet another tall order, but the good news is that there are myriad ways to make these things happen. So we start where we are, with whatever we've got on hand. Your previous training may or may not be helpful, your resources may or may not be adequate, your people might be all over the map with conflicting ideas about what to do and how to do it.

But no matter the details, you can think of your design as a bricolage experience, from the French verb *bricoler* ("to tinker"). As used in the world of arts and crafts, bricolage simply means working with whatever's handy: scraps of paper, tape, glue, organic materials, found objects, and so on. Lay it all out on the table and make something beautiful, or at least something interesting.

As an experiential designer, you can do likewise. Your facility isn't ideal, but you can make do. Your time available is too short, but you'll find a way. Your tech skills are minimal, but you'll get someone who can help. Your team is scattered, but you'll get them organized with a shared vision and a unifying narrative. It's going to be messy and it may not live up to your fantasy, but this is what you've got to work with. Objectives and utopian visions are valuable, but don't let the perfect be the enemy of the good. You've got work to do.

THE CREATIVE PATH

With this in mind, now would be a good time to look at some potential obstacles that might interfere and even cripple our creativity. In particular, we'd do well to be wary of the drama triangle, first described by psychologist Stephen Karpman in 1968. Often used as an explanatory tool in counseling and therapy, this model has powerful applications across the entire range of human experience, especially coaching, training, and teaching. Failure to heed the lessons of the drama triangle will have severe consequences for your people and your personal life.

According to Karpman, the trouble begins when a person identifies herself as a powerless victim in the face of circumstance. According to the victim's narrative, the source of her unhappiness lies with other people, agents, forces, and events. She pins the blame for her predicament on a persecutor or, if that doesn't work, she goes in search of a rescuer, someone or something that will extract her from her predicament and save the day.

Of course it's essential to remember there *are* genuine victims in this world; sometimes people are struck by lightning in one form or another through no fault of their own. Just as obviously, there are authentic persecutors and perpetrators who deserve justice. And absolutely, there are times when we can and should reach out to others for support; this need is a true human universal.

But the drama triangle is ultimately about our attitude, identity, and orientations. What role are we claiming in the world? Who is creating our lives? These are questions of agency, responsibility, and our relationship with the world at large.

The drama begins when we stumble, get hurt, or fail to get what we desire. Looking for a way out of our unhappiness, we label ourselves as victims. We blame our parents, our genes, our childhood, our jobs, our bosses, our associates, and our partners. We blame modern culture, government policy, the opposition party, stress, and overwork. To be sure, these accusations may well contain some elements of truth, but this is very much beside the point; the real issue is our orientation. By claiming the role of victim, we give away our power. No longer are we acting in the world—the world is acting on us.

Going to the other point of the triangle—toward rescue—is not much better. In our unhappiness, we look for people, substances, ideas, or organizations to bail us out of our predicament. But once again, we give away our power; the more we seek to be propped up by the world, the weaker we become. To be sure, support is a genuine human need and we are right to crave it, but beyond a certain point, we've got to stand on our own feet.

Many of us have heard this story before, and it's easy to assume that victimhood is something reserved for the dark underbelly of society; alcoholics, drug addicts, and criminals come to mind. But victimhood is alive and well at every level, and no one is immune. This includes everyone in the worlds of education and training: Teachers, coaches, trainers, students, clients, athletes are all vulnerable to the affliction.

But claiming victimhood is an easy, seductive trap that benefits no one. There's always plenty of blame to go around and excuses are always handy: The economy is in recession, our parents were flawed, our neighborhood was in turmoil. Bullies abused us, the schools failed us, the system didn't provide the kind of employment we deserved. In short, it's the world's fault that we're suffering. Accepting personal responsibility is simply out of the question. As victims everywhere put it, "It's not my job."

Not only does victimhood weaken our sense of power and agency, it's also bad for our health. When we see ourselves as powerless agents in a sea of influence, we simply go along with whatever lifestyle choices are presented to us. We lose contact with the strength and vitality of our primal bodies and hand our fate over to the forces of marketing, advertising, and corporate culture. When we cast ourselves as victims, we give up the very qualities that would protect us from adversity. Ultimately, adopting a victim orientation may be even worse for our health than widely recognized behaviors such as smoking and physical inactivity.

Even worse, the attitude is wickedly contagious, wreaking havoc on communities, organizations, schools, and teams. When people see us compulsively blaming perpetrators and running for rescue, the behavior soon becomes normalized. We come to believe that that's just how it's done in human society and, before long, everyone's working the drama triangle.

In turn, this sense of victimhood infects our politics and our culture, leading to the polarization and chaos we see today. That's why complaining has now become a national sport, with entire media empires dedicated to round-the-clock finger pointing. When things aren't going well, there's always a handy perpetrator we can blame, right across the aisle or down the street.

The way out of the drama triangle—as many educators, therapists, and coaches have suggested—is via the creative path. In other words, art. This is where we exercise responsibility and start building a vision of what we want to become. As we move beyond habits of blaming, complaining, excuses, and wishful thinking, life begins to open up into a world of opportunity, power, and freedom.

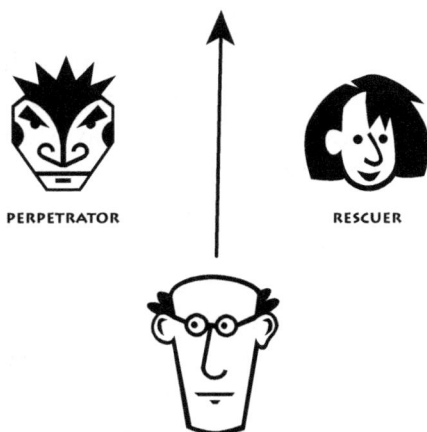

PERPETRATOR   RESCUER

In this practice, we actually change our identity. Instead of blaming circumstance or hoping for a rescue, we ask a new set of questions: What can I do today, right this moment, to advance my creation? Where can I exercise control? Where does my power lie? This is particularly vital for anyone who's working with experiential design.

In practice, teachers, coaches, therapists, and leaders must be on guard for drama and everything that goes with it. In particular, we need to create a culture of agency and responsibility. In this process, we discourage complaining and blaming, while we model action in the face of ambiguity and insecurity. We acknowledge pain, suffering, and trauma, and we seek out support when we need it; but no matter what, we keep our attention focused on our creation, whatever it might be.

Above all, this is the time to cultivate and nurture a creative orientation toward our work. Your experiential design must be *your* creation; it cannot be the mere repetition of a template or someone else's formula. Vital knowledge does exist and must inform our work, but ultimately, our interpretation and application must be a creative act. In this, our coaching, teaching, and leadership will always have more in common with art than any other profession. But instead of working with paint, clay, stone, or sound, we create with the experience of the human animal.

In this effort, we borrow a general principle from the world of sport and athletic training. As we'll see in later chapters, specific practice is the path to effective training and living. We learn precisely what we live; we become what we practice. We become more creative by exercising our creativity, we gain a stronger sense of agency by practicing agency, we get better at engaging with the world by engaging with the world. We get better at taking responsibility by taking responsibility.

Ultimately, being a teacher, trainer, or leader is all about our orientation. Yes, some predicaments are overwhelming and exhausting, and perpetrators must be called out. Likewise, we're right to reach out to one another when we're overwhelmed and in need of support. But no matter the depth of the adversity, we are free to choose our interpretations. We're free to choose our stories. We're free to move beyond complaining, blame, excuses, and rescue. The creative path is not an easy one, but this is where the meaning lies.

CHAPTER 3

ANCESTRY

If you don't understand the past, you won't have a future.

—Cherokee saying

Before digging deeper into the process of experiential design, we need to step back once again and ask some foundational, big-picture questions about the nature of the animals—the people—we're actually working with. If we get this wrong at the outset, we're going to be in a lot of trouble down the road, but if we get it right, we've got a chance to make a difference.

We're working with people, that much we can be sure of. But what exactly *are* people? Humans are so familiar to us that we scarcely even stop to think about what we really are, where we come from, or what we're doing with ourselves. People are our friends and family, our parents and children, our bosses and employees, our customers and our clients, our teachers and coaches. And for most of us, that's as far as our inquiry goes.

But when we set out to design effective experiences for our students, athletes, and clients, we'll never get far unless we understand what's going on inside their bodies, and in particular, the state of their nervous systems. And we'll never understand that until we understand their biological history, which is to say, their history as animals. So we begin with a quick review of who we are: vertebrates, mammals, primates, hominids, *Homo sapiens*.

BIG HUMAN HISTORY

The timeline is vast and the details are wickedly complex, but we can safely condense millions of years of history into a few paragraphs, starting with the geology and ecology of ancient Africa. If we were to travel back in time, tens of millions of years ago, we'd see that the entire continent was covered with dense forest. It was a haven for arboreal primates of all varieties; there was plenty of food in the trees, and it was easy to stay safe from predators. Life was good and the primates flourished.

Things might well have stayed that way except for a relatively sudden geologic event that opened up a substantial gap in East Africa, a feature now known as the Great Rift Valley. Tectonic plates shifted and, in turn, the regional climate became cooler and dryer, leading to a thinning of forest cover and the appearance of open grassland, a new ecological niche.

According to this so-called East Side Story, the new conditions created an open opportunity for bipedal primates who could travel more widely and exploit new food sources. Life wasn't always easy on the grassland, of course, and our ancestors were constantly faced with a host of ferocious predators. Nevertheless, they survived and even flourished, migrating in a series of overlapping diasporas, spreading the hominid and human lineages from Africa to Asia, Australia, and later to North and South America.

According to our best estimates, modern *Homo sapiens* have inhabited this planet for some 300,000 years, the vast majority of that time in primal, preagricultural conditions.

RADICAL COMMONALITY

From today's vantage point, it's easy to forget this story and, in particular, our radical commonality with all life on this planet. But like it or not, we are biological creatures and, in fact, all animal life on the planet is literally kin. The astonishing fact is that all of us—humans and every other life form on Earth—have descended from a single common ancestor, known as LUCA, the Last Universal Common Ancestor.

In all likelihood, LUCA was a simple microbial cell, similar to a modern bacterium. If we could play the movie of life backward, we would find LUCA at the starting point of a story that's been unfolding for almost four billion years. All living creatures on the planet are linked to this single-celled creature, the root of the tree of life.

The significance of LUCA is immense—scientifically, culturally, even spiritually. In short, LUCA unites us—or should unite us—via a story of shared origin and history. We may well behave otherwise, but we—the plants, animals, and humans of the biosphere—are truly, literally one. The entire history of life on earth is coursing through our veins in every minute of every day.

As a people, we have yet to fully appreciate the significance of LUCA, and it may be a long time before we integrate this understanding into our behavior and culture. Nevertheless, a sense of wonder is inescapable. Your body is not an arbitrary, isolated object that simply appeared on Earth. It's a leaf on an immense tree, a continuation of a process that is vast beyond our ability to comprehend. It's an amazing, awe-inspiring story. As Darwin himself put it, "There is grandeur in this view of life."

Likewise, humans have more in common with other primates than most of us would care to admit. We share similar physiologies, similar anatomies, and in particular, a similar genetic code. Anatomically and behaviorally, the differences between humans, chimpanzees, and bonobos are relatively minor. We live, eat, and socialize in ways that are sometimes almost indistinguishable. Modern people like to declare their independence from their animal cousins and from nature as a whole but, as zoologists and primatologists remind us again and again, the differences are almost insignificant and maybe even trivial.

Naturally, this radical commonality forces us to rethink our conventional approaches to almost everything, including and especially education, parenting, and coaching. And it also tells us a great deal about how we might envision our experiential design. In short, it suggests that we start treating people like animals.

If this proposition sounds odd, humorous, ironic, or preposterous, you might want to think again. This is a dead-serious proposal. Every veterinarian and dog trainer in the world understands how this works; humans are simply not that different. As mammals, we all have the same basic wiring and similar behavioral tendencies. Humans are unique in some ways, but every species has its unique features. It's also the case that our conventional approaches—treating people as independent agents, with no kinship with the natural world—have largely failed. Our epidemics of mental illness, distress, and discontent are stark reminders of that fact.

Instead, we need to think differently about our people and take their animal needs into account. It's no longer acceptable to treat people like "a brain on a stick," a passive receptacle for processing information. Instead, the time has come to see, feel, and appreciate our biological heritage, especially our perceptions of safety and danger.

In particular, we've got to respect our autonomic nervous systems and our stress responses. Just as with all mammals and primates, this system has powerful downstream consequences for physiology, learning, health, and behavior. If you can help your human animals feel felt and safe, you'll be well on your way to making them more receptive to learning and coaching. Respect the animal and things are going to go a lot better.

PARTICIPATORY CONSCIOUSNESS

Just as modern humans tend to forget their continuity with the natural world, we also largely ignore the presence, experience, and worldviews of native and indigenous people. Looking at the span of human and hominid history over the last several million years, it soon becomes obvious that modern society represents an incredibly recent, abrupt, and experimental development. We feel it as normal and familiar, but it's really an exception to our historically normal experience as hunters, gatherers, and nomads.

All of which forces us to ask a simple but vital question about humans and their behavior: What's normal for humans? What are the inclinations, attitudes, and worldviews that have animated people for most of our time on this planet? Obviously, there will be enormous diversity on this score; if there's one thing we know about humans it's that we're ferociously creative in building cultural solutions for survival. Nevertheless, anthropologists have identified a set of universal experiences and orientations that humans have shared throughout prehistory, which is to say, the vast majority of our time on Earth.

Most obvious, but often forgotten in today's world, is that ancient, historically normal humans lived extremely physical lives and were literally in touch with reality all day, every day. Hunting, gathering, and adventuring were routine activities and even back in camp, people were in constant contact with their bodies and sensations. There were no intervening devices or technologies to dilute the experience. Everyone in your tribe would have been athletic to some degree; survival depended on maintaining a robust relationship with our bodies.

But physicality was only a beginning. Our historically normal, ancestral experience was also marked by what's been called *participating consciousness*. That is, we lived inside nature and developed cultural practices that maintained and strengthened this continuity. In fact, ancestral people were keenly aware of their interdependence with the natural world—their bodies and spirits were permeable to life itself. There was no separation between mind and body or between body and habitat.

In fact, for native and indigenous people, identification with habitat has always been universal. "I am the land, the land is me." "I am the forest, the forest is me." "I am the river, the river is me." We hear these kinds of declarations in cultures all over the world, from Australia to Asia, Africa, and the Americas. It may sound jarring, alien, or quaint to modern ears, but for native people, this orientation is taken as self-evident, and there's nothing remarkable about it. In this respect, it is we—modern, disconnected urban dwellers—who are the outliers.

Going deeper, our ancestral experience was marked by *animism*, the belief and understanding that the whole world is alive. In modern terms, this orientation might be described as deep ecology or a biocentric philosophy. Indigenous humans never considered themselves superior; they saw themselves as equal participants in the vast drama of life. And far from being demeaning, there was comfort and even power in this view. When you're one with the most awesome force on the planet, the great drama of biological life, there's no limit to what's possible.

In turn, this indigenous, participatory worldview also inspired an ethical orientation that would serve us well in today's world. The three R's of the Cherokee tradition provide a typical moral code: relationality, responsibility, and reciprocity. When your very existence is interdependent with the biological world and the cosmos at large, you're naturally inclined toward this kind of humble, caring, and compassionate view. Far from being unusual in any way, this is the universal ethical philosophy for humanity; this is who we are.

In turn, this implies a tone and a value system for our experiential design. That is, we're not just delivering information or guiding people toward some kind of credential or achievement. We're actually trying to sustain an ethical tradition that's been in place for a very long time. By emphasizing humility, participation, responsibility, and reciprocity, we're positioning our children and clients for a deeper kind of success in relationship with the world at large. This orientation may well feel alien to you and your students, but it's actually the real status quo.

AWE

> Awe is the salve
> that will heal our eyes.
>
> —Rumi

Thinking about big human ancestry and our lives on the grasslands of East Africa, it's easy to dismiss the entire era as a grim, even gruesome battle for survival—a nasty, brutish, and short experience of deprivation and misery. But lost in our conversation is the fact that, in our intimate contact with nature, our lives would have been marked by an intense and captivating sense of awe.

Just imagine the enormity and immediacy of the experience; every day on the grassland would have been marked by thunderstorms, lightning displays, and animal dramas that played out in real time. With no light pollution, the night sky would have blazed with an intensity that modern humans can scarcely imagine. And around your tribe's local habitat, vast reaches of unknown territory stretched to the horizon, home to anything a person might imagine. In other words, awe was a daily experience. For hundreds of thousands of years, awe was routine.

But this experience was far more than a passive, feel-good nature show. Work by professor Dacher Keltner at UC Berkeley shows that even a mild sense of awe can change attitudes and inspire pro-social behavior. People who watched a nature video that elicited awe were subsequently more ethical and generous, and described themselves as being more connected to others—qualities that are commonplace in indigenous traditions. Keltner's team also found that awe makes people happier and less stressed, even weeks later. There's even a measurable health benefit.

A study by Jennifer E. Stellar and Neha John Henderson found that "positive emotions, especially awe, are associated with lower levels of proinflammatory cytokines."

Awe activates the parasympathetic nervous system, which works to calm the fight-flight response and dampen the production of toxic stress hormones. Awe also seems to help us break out of habitual thinking patterns as it improves creativity. In other words, putting ourselves in contact with nature's magnificence is really good for us. Research by psychologists at Stanford and the University of Minnesota has shown that awe can increase well-being by giving people a sense of "temporal affluence." We might even say that awe is a form of medicine.

Keltner and Jonathan Haidt have also argued that awe is the ultimate collective emotion because it motivates people to do things that enhance the greater good. Research reported in the Journal of Personality and Social Psychology provides empirical support for this claim. The authors found that awe helps bind us to others, motivating us to act in collaborative ways that enable strong groups and cohesive communities. Which, of course, is an ideal quality for both ancestral and modern life.

But for those of us who've grown up in narcissistic modern cultures, awe just doesn't get much attention or respect. Most of us like feeling big and celebrating our status as the alpha individuals or as part of the alpha species, but awe in natural settings does its work in reverse. It shrinks the ego and our sense of self, and in turn, leaves more space in our consciousness for the rest of creation. Incredibly, Keltner found that when test subjects were awe-inspired, they actually signed their names and drew themselves smaller. Other researchers have found that people who watched awe-inspiring videos estimated their bodies to be physically smaller than those who watched neutral videos.

All of which should give us pause. When we reflect on the radical differences between ancestral and modern life, we might well describe our modern condition as one of "awe deprivation" or an "awe vacuum." Today, fewer of us actually go outside, and when we do, most of our parks are highly domesticated, regulated, noisy, and light polluted. Our experience of awe—such as it is—mostly derives from our contact with gee-whiz technological devices and special effects in the movies we watch. This is massively reinforced by corporate marketing that attempts to attach our primal instincts to various products and services. In other words, our modern sense of awe, such as it is, is produced and managed—a plastic, manufactured imitation of the real thing.

Consequently, it's no surprise to find that our imagination has begun to atrophy. Disconnected from the wonders of wild animals, habitat, and the night sky, we lose our inspiration. Awash in synthetic narratives and artificial spectacle, we struggle to think for ourselves. Our imagination is weakening, crippled by the hypnotic qualities of our devices. Even worse, artificial intelligence now threatens to take control of our art, music, and language. But imagination is a muscle that atrophies with disuse, and as artificial awe comes to dominate our lives, human capacity will wither like a sedentary human body.

So what are we to do with the disappearance of awe in the modern human experience? Obviously, the ideal solution is to get more people back into intimate contact with big nature, vistas, panoramas, native plants, and animals. Far from being mere recreation or a pastime, this experience is absolutely vital to our welfare as a species and to our ability to create a functioning future. As it stands, some physicians are now enabled to write "green prescriptions" for their patients, but this just scratches the surface of what's necessary.

Of course, it would be a heavy lift to get millions of people out into the big outdoors, but we can also create a sense of awe through study, reading, and presentations. Teachers and coaches can tell the stories of big history and biology, not as conventional academic disciplines or as pathways to careers in biomedicine but as tools of psychospiritual awakening. Show your students the immensity of geologic and evolutionary time and the wonders of Darwin's "copiously branching bush." Astonish them with explanations of hypercomplex systems: human bodies, rainforests, oceans, and the cosmos at large. It's not a perfect solution by any means, and nothing really compares with direct contact with the ocean or the wild night sky, but there's awe and grandeur in this story as well.

FOCUS

When thinking about human prehistory, most of us are quick to think of hunting and gathering lifestyles, outdoor living, and our awe-inspiring exposure to the natural world. And we might even wonder about the knowledge, skill, and dexterity required to track animals, navigate, find water, and otherwise make a living in demanding conditions. But rarely mentioned in our conversations is the kind of focused attention that our ancestors must have enjoyed in daily life.

In a historically normal, Paleolithic setting, human attention must have been integrated and incredibly powerful; distraction was unheard of and monotasking was routine. Living in the semi-wooded mosaic grassland of East Africa, it was easy to hear and feel the primal signals coming from habitat and our bodies, and it was natural to pay attention to one thing at a time. Tracking an animal, watching the weather, talking with other people in your tribe; we could fully immerse ourselves in these experiences. Chip a stone tool, weave some fibers into a rope or a basket, build a fire, skin an animal—one integrated effort at a time. We were in flow almost every minute of every day. This was our normal state of consciousness.

But today we're faced with noise of a thousand varieties and our attention is under constant assault—in our cars, our homes, and even worse, our parks and natural spaces. Everyone wants a piece of us now, and our minds are fragmenting in the process. Attention spans shrink by the day as our consciousness becomes increasingly pixelated. As distraction machines, our devices contribute to an epidemic of loneliness, depression, and anxiety, especially in young people. Even worse, they displace basic human aptitudes such as navigation, conversation, and the exercise of judgment.

All of which creeps up on us little by little as we feverishly multitask our way through a world of cognitive overload and incessant homework. Overwhelmed by things that absolutely must be done, we compensate by going faster, by switching our attention rapidly from one task to another. And for a time, it seems to work. But as just about every neuroscientist in the world has told us, multitasking is a myth; the brain simply doesn't work that way. We focus, then shift, refocus, and shift again. In moderation, we can manage it, but over time, the process takes its toll in the form of exhaustion, error, and confusion.

The neuroscience is fascinating, but it's really just a confirmation of something that our elders have known for centuries. As the poet Publilius Syrus once quipped, "To do two things at once is to do neither." Likewise, an African parable tells us that "A good hunter does not chase two rabbits." And, as military strategist Sun Tzu surely would have put it, "To fight a dozen battles is to lose them all."

This is a powerful lesson for anyone working with experiential design. When setting up your program, drills, games, and activities, try to keep the focus on one challenge at a time. Likewise, it's safe to assume that the people who come to you are already in a state of multitasking overload. Their brains and their bodies are hyperkinetic and frenzied. Even worse, they might never have had an experience of deep immersion, flow, or mono-tasked engagement with the world. To put it bluntly, they don't even know what it feels like or why it might be important.

This is why stress-relief and relaxation exercises are so vital for our students, athletes, and clients. For people who are chronically afflicted by "the hurry disease," it can be very difficult to do anything else. And when the human animal is stressed, there's a very strong tendency to return to the familiar, which in this case is more of the same.

So look for ways to make relaxation a priority. We'll take a closer look at meditation in a later chapter, but for now, focus on focus. Encourage your people to concentrate on one thing at a time. Likewise, take a good look at your own style of concentration and what you're modeling. It's surely the case that attentional styles are contagious, and if you're constantly dividing your attention in a frenzy of multitasking, your people are sure to follow along.

CHAPTER 4

IS MY WORLD FRIENDLY?

A belief may be larger than a fact.

—Vannevar Bush

When we set out to train and develop high-functioning human animals, it's tempting to dive right into the process. We're eager to share our content, our experience, and our enthusiasms, so we jump into action, designing and executing our chosen programs and curriculums. But to create the magic we're seeking, there's some vital background work that we must do before we get started. In particular, it's essential that we come to an understanding of how the human animal experiences the world and how the body responds to the conditions it encounters.

How do people interpret reality and how do those interpretations drive behavior? How does the body manage its physiology and psychology in the face of ambiguous circumstances? In particular, how does it respond to perceived threats, danger, stress, and trauma?

These are big questions, but we can make a good start by considering another question, this one posed by the legendary physicist Albert Einstein. Sometime late in his career, a journalist asked if there was a fundamental question that people needed to ask about the nature of the Universe. The scientist famously replied, "I think the most important question facing humanity is, 'Is the universe a friendly place?'"

It was a great answer, not only for its cosmic implications, but for the fact that it aligns perfectly with what we now know about human neurobiology and brain function. As it turns out, humans and other mammals are asking this very same question from the time they're born and throughout their entire lives. The question runs in the background and is mostly unconscious, but it's elemental to our lives, our behavior, and our success or failure. In every moment our bodies wonder: "Is my habitat safe? Is my social world safe? What are my prospects for survival? Is my body going to be okay?"

In fact, the brain circuitry that drives this inquiry has been thoroughly mapped out. We now know that the amygdala serves as a sort of neurological radar or smoke detector, continuously alerting the rest of the brain and body to possible threats. This brain region, in conjunction with the limbic system and the cortex, gives us our assessments of danger and, in turn, helps drive our behavior. And in a very real sense, our entire life experience is primed and regulated by our answer to this primal inquiry. Whatever answer we come up with has very real neurological, health, and behavioral consequences—effects that reverberate throughout every minute of our lives and, in turn, throughout society at large.

Of course, it doesn't take much reflection to realize that our world is both friendly and unfriendly, and that wonders, pleasures, and comforts are all mixed up with threats, outright violence, chaos, and fear. If we look hard enough, we can find "evidence" for whatever answer we desire; humans are good at cherry-picking ideas and events that confirm our state of mind, body, and spirit.

To put it another way, our ultimate answer to this primal question will always be subjective, based on our history, our physiology, our character, our education, and our culture. In turn, our experiential design must take all this into account; how will our students, athletes, and children respond to a world that's both friendly and unfriendly?

COMPLICATIONS AND STRATEGIES

The challenge posed by the body's inquiry might seem simple enough, but there are plenty of complications. In the first place, our answer will be massively influenced by the disposition of the people around us. As hypersocial, tribal animals, we're extremely sensitive to the threat and danger assessments of the people we spend time with. Realize it or not, our bodies pay extremely close attention to the body language, posture, facial expressions, and tone of voice of people in our families and communities.

This isn't some vague whisper of intuition; it's rock-solid interpersonal neurobiology. If the people around us are feeling the friendliness of the world, we're likely to follow along, but if their bodies and language point to danger, we'll probably be swept up in the process. In other words, human danger assessments are extremely contagious, a process that's intimately familiar to anyone with experience in genuinely dangerous environments; for example, people involved in military operations and alpine climbing pay acute attention to the threat and danger assessments of partners and teammates.

Unfortunately, life in the modern world often gives us inconsistent, even neurotic answers to the friendliness question. Without a sense of shared predicament or a unifying narrative about who we are or where we're going, people around us may well be telling wildly different stories about the nature of the world at large. For some people, modern urban settings are easy to navigate and pose no particular threat; these people mostly remain in a comfortable state of rest-and-digest.

But for others, especially those who've suffered childhood trauma or poverty, the daily challenges of modern life can provoke a swift stress reaction. Naturally, people with a history of unfriendly experience are quick to assume unfriendliness in every encounter. All of which adds up to real social and physiological confusion; when the people around us are all on different autonomic pages, it's pretty hard to know what to do with our bodies and, in turn, our minds and our lives.

WHAT'S DANGEROUS?

Of course, if we happened to be living in a true Paleo environment, all of this would be much simpler. In your hunting and gathering tribe, everyone would have agreed on what's dangerous. Even children understand that lions and tigers and bears are hazardous, and there'd rarely be much confusion about the matter.

But in today's world, danger has gotten complicated. Every innovation carries the possibility of some new threat, and we're just not neurologically equipped to make these kinds of judgment calls. Real lions, real tigers, real bears—these creatures are easy to understand. But what are we to make of computer viruses, fine print in contracts, arcane rules, new devices, and novel substances that appear in our supermarkets and pharmacies?

And even worse, we largely fail to teach any of this. It's unlikely that you've ever taken a course called "An Introduction to Dangerous Things." As a result, our modern lives are marked by a creeping sense of foreboding and ambient fear. Surrounded by a new generation of vague threats, digital lions, bureaucratic tigers, and bad news bears, it's hard to know the truth. Is the world friendly? Who really knows? When in doubt, we assume the worst.

HAIR TRIGGER AND NEGATIVITY BIAS

A closely related complication is the hair trigger nature of our fight-flight system. In short, it's just easier to turn on a stress response. Calming down takes time, but we can fire up our fight-flight physiology in an instant. Naturally, this makes perfect sense in light of human evolution. After all, our Paleolithic homeland was a predator-rich environment and in this kind of setting, it pays to be a little bit paranoid and hypervigilant. If you see unfriendliness in some event and get it wrong, there's not much of a price to be paid, but err in the other direction and you might well be somebody's lunch.

This explains our negativity bias and tells us why—as psychologists put it— "the bad is stronger than the good." In essence, we're literally predisposed for vigilance and a touch of paranoia. This also explains why modern media is saturated with warnings of threat and danger; it's a proven method for capturing attention. If you want people to watch your show, make sure you scare them a little or maybe even a lot. Give them some lions and tigers and bears, real or imagined, and you'll capture some eyeballs.

LIONS, FAST AND SLOW

Another complication is something we might call the "slow carnivore problem." Again, this is easy to understand in terms of human evolution and our experience in ancestral environments. Just imagine a real-life lion coming into your camp; he's an immediate threat to you and your tribe right now, in this instant. Quite naturally, your autonomic nervous system goes on red alert and the entire neuroendocrine cascade goes into action. Likewise, everyone in your tribe will be primed to fight or flee. This is perfectly adaptive.

But now imagine some new species of slow predator, a giant but slothful beast that threatens to attack and demolish your camp in the future. What if our tribal shaman tells us to start worrying about an ominous creature that's coming for us several years from now? In this case, most of us will just shrug. Our brains just aren't primed for vigilance or action in response to threats that are distant in space and time. And even more to the point, we might not even be alive by then, so why worry?

This is why our response to the very real threats of climate chaos, biodiversity depletion, and looming agricultural failure have been so impotent. These threats are absolutely real and enormously consequential, but compared to immediate demands, they're rather slow moving and not so intimidating: We'll worry about those things later, if at all. This also suggests that, if we're going to be persuasive about these threats, we'll have to increase our sense of urgency and make the dangers more vivid in the popular imagination.

STRESS EFFECTS

Not surprisingly, stress also has a lot to do with how we answer our question about the friendliness of the world. Obviously, the more acute and chronic the stress, the more likely people will be to see the world as unfriendly. But this is more than just a psychological reaction or inclination; it's a profoundly biological process. Stress can even be passed down to a fetus in the womb, as stress hormones circulate in the mother's body, shaping the early development of key brain structures such as the amygdala, the hippocampus, and the prefrontal cortex. Yes, it's true—some of us are actually born into the world primed for danger and unfriendliness.

It's also the case that the way we answer the friendly question will have extended, long-range consequences for our bodies, our relationships, and our health. Suppose you hold the belief that your world is fundamentally unfriendly. If that's the case, you're likely to see threats in every direction and you might even hold a defensive stance or psychologically armor your body against anticipated trauma. This might be appropriate in the short term, but chronic psychophysical defense takes its toll on our health and might even contribute to illness along the way.

But if your answer is "Yes, the world is usually friendly," your stance and body posture will be more welcoming in anticipation of likely pleasures. A more welcoming body is less guarded, more pliable, and more receptive to the world at large. All of which contribute to better physiological function and health. Even better, you're more likely to seize opportunities that come your way in life.

In any case, our experience tends to be sticky and enduring, especially when it's stressful and traumatic. Survival is always the first priority for the body, and having a vivid memory of life-threatening events is sure to serve us well in the event of similar experiences in the future. When trauma comes at us and support fails, the body makes a reasonable prediction: Future conditions are likely to be similarly dangerous and incoherent. To put it another way, trauma and stress aren't one-off events that come and go with the wind, and we can't just shake them off and carry on as if nothing happened. Rather, these events leave lasting impressions on the nervous system; they are over-learned, over-remembered, and stored in the body.

MATCHES AND MISMATCHES

So here's the tricky part of all of this: If our answer to the friendly question matches actual conditions in habitat and the world at large, we're in good shape. If we're inclined to friendliness in a world that's actually friendly, all goes well. Or if we're on guard and vigilant in a world that's truly dangerous, we'll at least be mostly safe.

But if our stories and actual conditions are out of sync, things get problematic in a hurry and it's easy to see difficulties in both directions. Holding a soft, welcoming, and receptive attitude in a genuinely dangerous world is a recipe for disaster; lions and tigers and bears might literally have you for lunch. Conversely, holding a hypervigilant and hair-trigger attitude in a setting that's actually nurturing is a formula for overreaction, bad judgment, ruined relationships, and catastrophic career moves.

Of course, the stories we tell about the friendliness of the world are massively influenced by our early childhood experiences, even in utero, for better or for worse. Children are acutely aware of the danger assessments of their elders, and in turn, this experience is reflected in the biology and physiology of their bodies.

This adds up to a vital insight. That is, the way your parents and elders answered the "friendly" question is likely to be the way you'll answer it as well, even years and decades later. There's even a good chance that you'll pass a similar answer down to your children and the people around you, either explicitly or unconsciously, by way of your attention, stories, and behavior.

This all makes good sense, but sadly, our personal narratives about the ultimate nature of the world are often displaced and eclipsed by the synthetic commercial narratives that have come to dominate modern consciousness. The problem with synthetic narratives is that they don't just lure us into buying particular products and services; they also manipulate our perceptions of safety, security, and friendliness.

In the context of human history, this kind of storytelling is wickedly abnormal. In fact, today's synthetic narratives are so far removed from their original, organic form that they're best described as "plastic narratives" or "narrative products." Like highly refined food products, these narratives are distilled and stripped of their original nutrients and meaning. They're intentionally produced not to reveal, express, or enlighten but to manipulate and exploit.

But just as excess consumption of food products eventually compromises our health, the chronic consumption of synthetic narratives ultimately degrades our ability to think clearly about danger and friendliness. Narrative products sound like real stories and are highly palatable, maybe even tastier than the real thing, but the danger is real to individuals and our culture as a whole. Try to get by on a diet of synthetic narratives and you'll eventually lose contact with your identity, your history, and your purpose.

All of which leads us to the crux of the matter. That is, our challenge is to craft personal and collective narratives that fit actual conditions on the ground; appropriate and accurate stories about the friendliness and unfriendliness of the world. Likewise, this suggests a specific role and job description for every leader, teacher, trainer, coach, and parent. That is, we aren't just teaching particular skills or disciplines; we're also helping people fine-tune their understandings of the world.

So help your people focus their attention and relinquish their concerns about false tigers. Don't let them get distracted by the overhyped, often imaginary threats that pour into their lives via the digital firehose. If you can help your people concentrate on real tigers and truly authentic dangers, they've got a much better chance of surviving and thriving into the future.

All of which leads us to the most crucial challenge of all: the ability to maintain our equipoise, even in the face of genuinely unfriendly forces and events. As most of us know by personal experience, perceptions of stress and danger can be extremely corrosive to our performance. As the unfriendliness closes in, our bodies contract and our minds begin to seize up; we lose our physical fluency, our athleticism, our equanimity, and in the extreme, even our humanity itself.

The solution of course, is training and practice, especially in challenging but supportive circumstances. When a stressful experience becomes familiar, it loses its power to hijack our brains and bodies; we've been there before and survived. The encounter may still be stressful in some degree, but we'll have confidence, based on our actual lived experience. In this sense, our lived success becomes an antidote to the panic and paralysis that comes with stress and danger.

As a teacher, coach, parent, or leader, look for ways to incorporate this understanding into your experiential design. Ideally, the challenges you create will be precise and specific to actual experiences that your students, athletes, and clients will encounter, but it's also true that *any* form of challenging experience can have an inoculating, calming effect. Present your people with an experience that's slightly unfriendly and give them support as they fight their way through it. This will serve them well next time they encounter the lions, tigers, and bears in their lives. They've succeeded before and they can do it again.

IS MY WORLD COHERENT?

Our answer to the friendliness question is fundamental to the human experience, but there's also a similar set of questions that will help us fine tune our inquiry: "Is my world coherent?" "Is reality reliable?" "Can my world be trusted?"

This is the approach taken by Aaron Antonovsky, an Israeli-American sociologist and academic who studied Holocaust survivors and the relationship between stress, health, and well-being. A rebel and an idealist, Antonovsky also pioneered the concept of *salutogenesis*, the idea that certain experiences are vital in the upstream creation of health. After years of research, Antonovsky came to the conclusion that the key ingredient in human health and adaptation is not the familiar formula of diet and exercise, but rather the psychological experience of *coherence*.

In the most general sense, coherence is a state or situation in which parts or ideas fit together so that they form a united whole. But Antonovsky went further, suggesting that salutogenic, health-promoting experiences should be *comprehensible*, *controllable*, and *meaningful*. The beauty of this approach is that it gets to the psychophysical root of our experience, our suffering, and even our success in dealing with the world.

When we feel that the world is coherent, predictable, and reliable, our brains and our bodies relax. We understand our conditions, we can control them to some degree, and we feel that our efforts matter. For Antonovsky, this is the core of the entire human enterprise. When we feel that reality is reliable, trustworthy, and predictable, our stress-response system calms down and we ease into a more relaxed frame of being. In turn, this allows the body's natural healing processes to take over.

In contrast, taking away people's sense of coherence is profoundly destructive, even debilitating. This might be the inadvertent consequence of poorly managed programs and institutions, but in some cases it's darkly intentional. This is what we see in gritty spy novels that describe brutal interrogation procedures in secret black ops sites. When intelligence agencies attempt to coerce prisoners into revealing information, their first priority is to destroy their prisoner's sense of coherence. Make reality unreliable, take away familiar patterns of light and dark, food and social contact, trust and predictability. In short, make the experience as random and fragmented as possible. In the extreme, this experience terrorizes the prisoner and, in theory, causes him to give up valuable information.

Which naturally begs the question: What of our

experience in the modern world? Is it coherent? Is reality reliable or unreliable? Can we depend on things being relatively stable and predictable? Are conditions comprehensible, controllable, and meaningful? Can we relax? Can we trust?

The short answer is that, whatever the ultimate nature of modern social reality, there's no denying that many of us feel that the world is increasingly incoherent, unstable, and unreliable. There's no unifying narrative to guide our efforts, no unified culture or leadership, no clear vision of where we're going or what we're doing on this planet; it just feels like "shit happens." And not only does the world feel incoherent today, it's threatening to become even more so in the years and decades to come.

The causes of this incoherence are obvious: runaway computing technology, the Internet, social media, invasive marketing, and in particular, rogue political leaders who play fast and loose with the conventional norms, institutions, and sacred values that hold society together. Like prisoners in a black ops site, we're suffering under a jarring stream of disconnected stimuli, and even worse, digital media functions as a kind of incoherence machine, breaking our understanding into pieces and driving our angst around the clock. And it's this incoherence, even more than a poor diet or sedentary living, that poses the greatest threat to the well-being of the modern human animal.

Of course, the level of coherence or incoherence we experience depends a great deal on our social class, rank, and social relationships. For the affluent, it's pretty easy to view the world as stable and reliable. If you've got the money, you can bend reality to your will and your experience will be more coherent, predictable, and friendly. So yes, you can relax and your mind-body will work better. In turn, you can build even more coherence into your world and enjoy the process as it unfolds.

But for those in poverty, the answer is an unequivocal *no*. Without financial power or resources, the world becomes increasingly incoherent, unreliable, unpredictable, and unstable. It's not simply that poor people have less money; the world that they're living in is altogether different—more threatening, more dangerous, more random, less predictable, and more stressful. It's no surprise that their health suffers.

That said, there's more to this process than money and political power. When it comes to building and maintaining a sense of coherence, social relationships can make or break our efforts. It's easy to see how this might work in teams, families, and the workplace. Just like our sense of danger, our sense of coherence is also contagious. If the people around us are experiencing the world as reliable, predictable, and stable, they'll naturally radiate an infectious sense of ease, and friends, neighbors, and coworkers will respond in kind.

But when the people around us feel the world as incoherent, tensions will rise, paving the way for increased fear, xenophobia, toxic tribalism, and yet more incoherence. In other words, the cascades and ripple effects are very real and extremely consequential.

PRESCRIPTIONS

Antonovsky's teachings are immensely valuable for anyone working with experiential design, and we'd do well to keep coherence in mind when putting our programs into action. Even better, they also dovetail with the insights of modern stress science. The work of neurobiologist Robert Sapolsky is particularly useful in this regard. Writing in *Scientific American* in December 2005, Sapolsky summed up the research-based findings this way:

> Individuals are more likely to activate a stress response and are more at risk for a stress-sensitive disease if they...
>
> - feel as if they have minimal control.
> - feel as if they have no predictive information.
> - have few outlets for their frustration.
> - lack social support.

The beauty of this list is that it gives us a simple guide for creating experiential designs that ease the stress on the human animal and, in turn, set the stage for learning, creativity and function. Just follow the list:

> Give people a sense of **control** in whatever way you can. Give them progressive challenges that they can master, gaining control over their bodies and the skills in question. Look for things that people can actually do, and do better. Even the completion of simple tasks adds to a sense of mastery. Agency and engagement are key.

> Give people a sense of **predictability**. Tell them what's coming up today, tomorrow, next week, next month. Avoid random or arbitrary challenges unless there's a compelling reason to do so. Allow people to metabolize new information before you add

additional challenges.

Give people **outlets** for whatever frustration they might be experiencing. Physical movement is the most obvious example; even short movement snacks give people the chance to shake off their stress and express what they're feeling. Social expression and conversation can have a similar effect.

Above all, give people **social support**. Model supportive behaviors and make it clear that support is an implicit part of your culture; everyone in your program is responsible for everyone else.

Likewise, we can follow Antonovsky's lead in our crafting our experiential designs:

Make your programs **comprehensible**. Will your patients, students, or athletes understand your objectives and the challenges you put before them? Are you clear in what you're asking people to do?

Make the experience **controllable**. Are your activities within the grasp of your students or athletes? Even if the skills themselves are temporarily out of reach, is the overall experience something that your people can manage? Will they feel the potential for mastery?

Make the experience **meaningful**. Is your program relevant to people's lives in some significant way? Does it connect to any larger social, ecological, or personal issues? Does it hold some promise beyond a certificate or credential? Is it more than just a bunch of information? Does it connect to the lived experience of your people?

Like any good story, there should be an arc to the challenges and curriculum, a progression, a theme, and a trajectory. Give people a sense of where they are and where they're going. Don't be afraid to repeat yourself. "This is what we're doing and why we're doing it." "Here's what's coming." And most important of all, "This is how it relates to the rest of your life."

TRAUMA-INFORMED

Just as your students, clients, and athletes live in world that often feels incoherent, unpredictable, and unreliable, it's also the case that many of us—even most of us— will have some prior experience with trauma in our lives. Far from being a rare or unusual event, many of us are now beginning to realize that trauma is actually commonplace, if not ubiquitous, across the modern world.

This understanding has been brought to popular attention by physician and author Gabor Maté. From Maté's view, the modern world is inherently stressogenic and often traumatizing. As we saw in our conversation about mismatch, the human animal is fundamentally out of sync with modern conditions and sadly, we fail to see just how problematic our situation really is. Like frogs in warming water, we keep adapting and telling ourselves that the problem lies with us, not with the world at large. Something is wrong with our individual brains perhaps; maybe our neurotransmitter levels are out of order or maybe we just need to adjust.

But this is a fundamental misunderstanding of our situation. As Maté puts it: "The myth of normal is that we assume the conditions of society are healthy simply because we're used to them." This belief is extremely problematic because it blinds us to the true nature and pathology of our predicament. Instead of taking political action on large-scale systems, we blame ourselves.

Likewise, Maté teaches us that trauma isn't just in our heads. Rather, it lives in our bodies, in our nervous systems, keeping us stuck in a survival mode of perpetual fight, flight, freeze, or fawn. We feel numb and exhausted, we overthink everything, we drive toward perfection, or we push others away. Hypervigilant for anything that reminds our bodies of the original insult, we live our lives on edge. Even worse, this is not simply an issue for affected, traumatized individuals themselves. Our stress and trauma responses are highly contagious, rippling through society and culture, ratcheting up our tension and anxiety, even if we're not directly affected.

As for the origin story behind our trauma, Maté points to three vital experiences that the human animal must have to live a healthy and fulfilling life. If any of these elements are missing, thriving becomes more difficult.

Secure attachment is the first essential. Born helpless and incompetent into an unknown world, the human infant must bond to a caregiver, someone who stands ready to protect us from a wild and unknown world. When we feel felt by someone, the body relaxes and begins to devote its resources to growth and development. In turn, we feel comfortable; we've got a safe home base from which we can go out and explore the world. But if attachment fails, the infant is forced to navigate a world far beyond its powers; the result is stress that can linger throughout life.

As we grow into adulthood, we also feel the need for a sense of **agency and authenticity**, the sense that we can do things in the world, that we can master our lives with a sense of control over our circumstances. We feel a craving to become who we want to be, but if agency and authenticity are denied, we languish as partially formed beings, never reaching our strength or potential. In the process, we become vulnerable to any passing stresses that might confront us later in life.

Maté teaches us a great deal about trauma and healing, but his most important call is for a more trauma-informed society. In other words, we can no longer assume that trauma is a rare or exceptional event. Major institutions, governments, organizations, and policies should explicitly integrate this new understanding into practice. Going further, we might also call for trauma-informed medicine, trauma-informed government, trauma-informed education, and trauma-informed leadership. Since trauma touches every corner of society, every institution and system needs to be aware and involved.

Naturally, this includes our work as coaches and teachers. Whatever kind of experiences we create for our students, clients, or athletes, they should always be trauma-informed and trauma-aware. We may not be able to provide direct care for individuals, but at the very least, we must be aware of the possibility, even the likelihood, that the people we're working with have suffered and are continuing to suffer. In other words, it's safe to assume trauma, or at least the possibility of trauma, in everyone who participates in our programs.

THE BOTTOM-UP APPROACH

When working with stressed or traumatized human animals, one of the most powerful strategies is to start with the body. This is the recommendation of Bessel van der Kolk, author of the bestselling *The Body Keeps Score*. In short, he describes three pathways to healing:

The first is the familiar, "top down" cognitive approach that relies heavily on language, narrative, and explanation. Talk therapy is an obvious example, but we also see this kind of approach in informal settings where we use conversation to re-frame one another's experience and provide explanations for why things are the way they are.

The second pathway is biomedical and includes all manner of substances, medicines, and technological interventions, all of which are aimed at tissues, metabolism, physiology, neurotransmitters, and genes.

Both these methods have value, but for Van der Kolk, the third pathway is where the real action is. This is the "bottom-up," somatic, experiential approach, an orientation that holds immense promise, especially for those who've suffered trauma, chronic stress, or deep adversity over long periods of time. In other words, words might be useful, but ultimately, the body needs *experiential proof* that the world is in fact a friendly place. As Van der Kolk puts it, "All trauma is preverbal." No amount of language, no matter how eloquent, will substitute. The body wants to know the nature of its world, and it's our job to show them. Our job is to make a case, not to the mind but to the whole organism. In fact, what Van der Kolk is proposing is nothing less than a form of experiential medicine.

In the world of therapy and counseling, this approach is gaining wider acceptance as more and more people come to appreciate the power of the body in creating our mental states. But how do we make it work?

You may not be a therapist and you're probably working

with diverse groups of people. Some of your students, clients, or athletes are suffering lingering trauma, some are merely stressed, and others are doing pretty well. How do we contradict the helplessness, rage, and collapse that our people have experienced in the past?

There can be no single formula, and there are surely thousands of ways to give people the experiential proof that they need. Much will depend on your history, methods, and personal style. But all of that aside, we might do well to adopt a veterinary model, which is to say again, yes, treat people like animals. How would you treat a group of nonhuman animals who've been traumatized or stressed? What kind of culture or experience would you create? Can you contradict their history of trauma and stress?

Conceptually at least, this should be easy. Your students, clients, athletes, and patients have the same basic wiring and stress-responsiveness as any other mammal. When we experience a "perceived threat to the organism" as the stress scientists put it, we fire the same brain regions, and stimulate the same kind of glands, with similar hormones that have similar effects on health, disposition, and experience. Likewise, the experiential proof that we're looking for should be substantially the same if not outright identical: predictability, coherence, compassion, time, and above all, a sense of "feeling felt." Ask any dog trainer; what works for the skittish rescue dog should also work for your skittish students, athletes, clients, and patients.

TRIBE OR DIE

As most everyone knows, our answer to the friendliness question also has a great deal to do with how we see ourselves in relationship to our various tribes, teams, and communities. As hypersocial animals, tribe has historically functioned as a true life-support system and it's easy to see why. Just imagine yourself living in an ancestral environment, exposed and vulnerable on the semi-wooded grassland of East Africa, any time in the last several hundred thousand years. In this setting, there's really nothing between you and the carnivorous beasts that prowl just outside your camp. To put it in modern terms, you're living in a predator-rich environment.

In this setting, staying alive is a daily priority and the only thing between you and the claws and teeth of the big cats is your ability to gang up and stick together. There's no going it alone, not for long anyway; isolation would be a death sentence. So you've got to stay with your people and present a united front against your adversaries. And not surprisingly, you'll develop extreme social sensitivity to any social signals of inclusion and exclusion. Your people are the only thing standing between you and a miserable, terrifying death; of course you'll pay attention to how you're being treated by others.

Over time, this hyper-sensitive social awareness has literally been written into our brains and incorporated into the deepest layers of our bodies. The brain is very much a social organ and much of our circuitry is devoted to monitoring, tracking, and adjusting our relationships with one another. In fact, we use much of the same neural circuitry to process physical pain and the pain of social rejection; breakups don't just hurt in a psycho-romantic way, they *actually* hurt. And conversely, performing acts of altruism activates reward centers in the brain; doing good for other people literally feels good.

Now, multiply this need for social affiliation across

thousands of generations of hunter-gatherers and suddenly, things become clear. Our ancient vigilance remains and impacts much of our modern social experience, even in the absence of immediate danger. The big cats no longer stalk us, but we still feel the same sense of exposure as our ancestors. Even as we've exterminated most of the predators on the planet, our minds continue to evaluate our social standing relentlessly.

It may not be obvious, especially when conditions are friendly, but all of us continue to live on the crux between acceptance and rejection, inclusion and exclusion, affiliation and banishment in every moment of every day. No matter our situation, we remain hypersensitive to any clues that might tell us whether or not we're invited to the party.

But this is where it gets messy. All of us belong to multiple social groups and perceive our social standing differently. Some of your students, clients, and athletes will feel secure in their community affiliation, but others will be living on the social edge, terrified of rejection and exclusion. And somehow, you've got to get all these people working together within the context of your experiential design.

Naturally, this is an art in itself, but it all begins with our willingness to slow down and emphasize humanity and inclusion. Make sure that all of your students, clients, and athletes feel welcome, accepted, and needed. Frequent reminders of unity and shared predicament will go a long way. You may not have big carnivores prowling the perimeter of your program, but the need for unity remains.

LIFE IN THE BOWL

As experiential designers, our goal is to create something that supports the learning process and the spirit of the human animal. As we all know, people learn better when they believe that the world is friendly. Their nervous systems relax, they're less vigilant and defensive, and they're more curious and creative. This is the ideal condition.

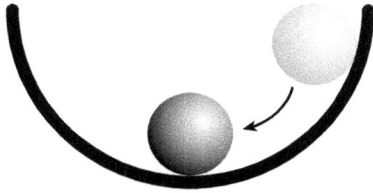

To understand this psychology in the simplest possible way, let's borrow a simple metaphor from the world of physics and engineering. Just imagine two conditions involving a ball and a bowl. When we place the ball inside the bowl, we create a condition of positive stability. The ball can move, but the shape of the bowl will guide it back toward the center. This is an ideal state for any complex system, from atmospheres to bioregions, from physiology to psychology. The sides of the bowl constrain and regulate the movement, and guide it back to homeostasis.

Now consider the inverse. Take the bowl, turn it upside down, and place the ball on top. Naturally, this becomes a case of negative stability; if the ball moves by even a small amount, the shape of the bowl will lead it further and further away from safety. Almost instantly, this becomes a runaway state of acceleration and, ultimately, disaster.

Obviously, this describes many of our systems in the modern world, most notoriously the dynamics of our atmosphere and the biosphere. As regulation fails and feedback processes kick in, change accelerates, leading ultimately to chaos and collapse. The same metaphor also applies in the worlds of physiology, society and economics; without some form of regulation, dynamic systems are doomed to failure.

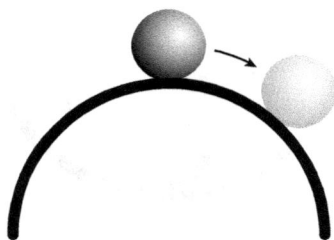

The ball-and-bowl metaphor tells us a great deal about human psychology and in particular, how it feels to live in modern society. If the human animal perceives herself to be a ball inside a life-supporting social and cultural bowl, all is well. She can move around, play, experiment, and make mistakes in her relationships and career, but the walls of the bowl—the people, rituals, and institutions around her—will gently guide her back to the center.

As a consequence, she feels safe. She can face the ambiguity of the world without undue fear; if she screws up, the bowl will be there to get her back to equanimity and balance. Life inside a bowl is not just safer, it's healthier and more sustainable.

But when we feel like we're perched on top of an inverted social or cultural bowl, everything goes the other way. At the very least, we're going to feel uneasy, anxious, stressed, and vulnerable. The world doesn't feel friendly in the slightest. We have no sense of safety, no means of support, and most of all, we feel exposed. If we do everything perfectly, we might be okay, but if we want to play, experiment, or take risks, there will be nothing between us and oblivion. No wonder we feel edgy and apprehensive; one false move and you're a goner.

All of which tells us a great deal about modern society and our experiential design efforts. Are people living in the bowl or on top of an inverted bowl? Judging by our deteriorating mental health and escalating levels of anxiety, stress, and depression, it's safe to assume that society is becoming inverted. Most humans are living in jeopardy now, with the threat of disaster looming in every moment. If we make a mistake, get something wrong, fail to get the job, fail to secure affordable housing, or fail to get into the right social network, we may well fall off the edge and into economic and psychosocial ruin.

This also points to a fundamental difference between native and modern cultures. Indigenous people have long understood the need for supporting structure, rituals, and experiences. Community is the bowl, and when people value community, they're keeping that vital sense of stability alive. In fact, the people of Guinea, West Africa even have a word describing a safe place or place of refuge: *kissidugu*. These people understand how humans work in society; when we support community, we're really supporting ourselves.

In contrast, modern society is upside down. In our hypercompetitive, radically independent culture, many of us are effectively on our own. And for free-market zealots, this is precisely as it should be. There's no need for social services, no need to regulate the dynamics of complex systems, no need to support people in need. According to this narrative, the invisible hand of the market will magically take care of everything.

But the consequences of such an orientation are perverse: The affluent live like a ball in a supporting bowl, but for everyone else, it's a precarious, tenuous, fragile, and even terrifying existence. And if you happen to fall off the side of the bowl, that's on you.

All of which speaks volumes for our experiential design. In the first place, it's safe to assume that many of your students, clients, and athletes will have some sense of living on top of the inverted bowl. They may be performing adequately at the moment, but the abyss is never far away, and they're sure to feel this predicament in their bodies.

With this in mind, we look for ways to create conditions of support. You can build the walls of the bowl with policies and procedures, but ultimately, the most powerful approach is human. That is, we give people a sense of comfort and security by slowing down, paying attention to their experience, and above all, building trust with consistent communication. When people make errors or get off track, guide them back to the center where they can relax and try again.

FEELING FELT

In all likelihood, you won't be able to do much about the large-scale public or economic policy decisions that make people feel like they're perched precariously on top of an inverted bowl, but we can make our programs personally supportive. We do this with rituals, games, and culture, but mostly we do it with time and personal attention.

Unfortunately, this may well feel like an uphill battle in a world where commercial and professional encounters are dominated by short, superficial relationships. Time is expensive, we believe, and we're in a hurry to do the transaction, whatever it is. We're trying to be efficient, but humanity takes time, so we skip over the casual talk, the gossip and the personal stories that bond us together. We get straight to the point and get the work done, but in the end, these short encounters leave people feeling marooned, isolated, alienated, and even manipulated. Our bodies want to connect, but there's just no time, so we're forced to find our humanity elsewhere.

But our students, athletes, and clients have a deep-seated desire to feel seen, heard, felt, understood, respected, and appreciated. This need is a true human universal. People of every age, culture, origin, and status need and crave this experience. Even the Na'vi, the indigenous people of Pandora depicted in the movie Avatar, address one another with the honorific "I see you."

This need for basic recognition is not a "nice to have" experience nor is it a superficial "frosting on the cake" to be layered on top of other content or educational experiences. This is a powerful biological drive that goes all the way to the deepest levels of physiology and nervous system function. In other words, our need to feel felt is as real as our need for food and water. When the body feels recognized and appreciated, the autonomic nervous system goes into action, repairing tissues and opening up our cognition and creativity. Without question, this experience is a powerful and inexpensive form of medicine in its own right.

But sadly, the experience of feeling felt, heard, seen, respected, and appreciated is rapidly disappearing from our modern cultural landscape. In the very domains where we would most desire and expect it—education and medicine—it's often absent, eclipsed by administrative and technical urgencies. As we race from one task to another, our communications become increasingly superficial and we neglect this fundamental human need. Tragically, many students, clients, and patients go years without feeling felt, and some of us never experience it at all.

As a culture, we've lost sight of the primal, human fundamentals. Perversely, we take something that is (or was) intrinsically human and professionalize it. We wrap it up in technical language and hand it over to an expert class of psychologists and therapists. Today, if you really want to feel felt, you might have to pay an expert to do something that an average, nonexpert human should be able to do without any training whatsoever. This professionalization of our humanity is sometimes presented as a solution to our mental and spiritual distress, but it's really a reflection of our alienation and our failure to master the fundamentals of being good social animals.

For teachers, coaches, therapists, and parents, this all comes down to a simple question: "Do my people feel felt, heard, seen, appreciated, and respected?" This is the gold standard in evaluating personal and professional relationships. In turn, we give these qualities to others as often as possible, to everyone in our world. This is a primal interpersonal gift, far more valuable and consequential than any physical object. When we take the time to see, hear, and recognize one another, we're actually giving a gift to their bodies and their lives. We're giving them medicine.

To put this another way, what we're looking for in leadership is rich communication, bringing the totality of our attention to bear on our conversations, our relationships, and our interactions. This means being completely present and setting aside our distractions, for the time being at least. The practice demands time, sincerity, and a willingness to stick with the encounter as it unfolds. We communicate safety by slowing down and giving our conversations and bodies some room to breathe. This adds up to a more expansive experience for everyone involved.

Of course, this rich communication is a discipline, and some would call it a dying art. Every time we speed up or divide our social and conversational attention into multiple tracks, we create anxiety and disconnection in ourselves and our listeners. People don't feel heard and when they don't feel heard, they're more likely to wonder about our true intentions. And even worse, their attention will begin to fragment, leading to a runaway collapse of communication and, possibly, the entire relationship.

Practically speaking, we can't practice rich communication in every social encounter, but we can develop our capability by following the athletic model for specific training. That is, we get proficient at something by practicing that very thing. We get better at rich communication by practicing rich communication. We get better at slowing down by actually slowing down and fully inhabiting our conversations and our interactions. So stop thinking about transactions and start paying attention to the animal in front of you. This is where the real action is.

CHAPTER 5

HOW WE LEARN

The eight laws of learning are explanation,
demonstration, imitation, repetition, repetition,
repetition, repetition, repetition.

—John Wooden

I was an ordinary person who studied hard.
There are no miracle people.

—Richard Feynman

When we set out to transform our athletes, students, or children into high-functioning human animals, we've got to develop an understanding of how people actually learn the world. It's tempting to simply follow along with the programs and methods given to us by tradition, but our understanding of neuroscience has changed radically over the last few decades, and we've come to realize that a lot of our conventional methods are inefficient at best and counterproductive at worst.

This new understanding will give us some powerful lessons, but before we get to the details, it's essential that we review a short history of education itself.

OLD SCHOOL

We begin with the most fundamental human learning experience of all, that of our hunting and gathering ancestors, but right away we're faced with a bit of a surprise, even a shock. That is, most of us don't even think about hunters and gatherers as learners at all. According to our cartoon stereotype, there simply was no education on the grassland of East Africa. Our ancestors simply survived in the bush, eking out a desperate living as they fought back against wild animals, bad weather, and assaults by neighboring tribes. These people weren't students or scholars, they were nothing more than ignorant brutes. Rarely if ever do we think of them as intelligent, sophisticated, educated, or cultured.

But in fact, our ancestors were extremely competent learners and scholars of the natural world. They had to be. Just imagine the depth and breadth of what a young person would need to know to survive and thrive on the grassland: the behaviors of plants and animals and how they interacted, how to follow tracks, how to prepare food, how to understand the weather and the seasons, how to build fire and prepare poison-tipped arrows.

In fact, this body of knowledge would have been immense, all of it built with the same neurological capabilities we use today. And arguably, the educational engagement of hunter-gatherers was actually *more* robust than that of the most rigorous modern, academic institutions. These people learned deeply because their lives depended on it. They learned because they lived it.

Of course, our original hunter-gather education was based entirely on lived, physical experience in habitat. The process was intimate, personal, emotional, and subjective.

There were no books, no classrooms, no lectures, no gyms, no clinics, no lesson plans. Not only was this kind of training historically normal, it was also incredibly successful and, in contrast with modern pedagogies, it's a proven method. To put it another way, experiential education has been the status quo for 99.9 percent of our time on the planet. We're here today, not because of our academic training in modern schools, but because of the experiential learning of those who came before us.

It's not difficult to imagine how this process might have unfolded in a typical indigenous or Paleolithic camp. As a child, you would have watched adults leave camp on hunting excursions, returning home with stories about their adventures and encounters with animals, weather, and terrain. You would have heard from gatherers who foraged the perimeter of camp and found water or medicinal herbs. Excited to learn more, you were eager to follow along and learn about the world.

In this process, sensation and attentional training would have been fundamental. Working exclusively in an oral tradition, elders would have told young people, "Look here. Smell this, taste this. Notice the way that the animal tracks in the riverbed go this way, then that. Notice how the hunters sometimes go fast, then go slow. Sometimes we chase, but sometimes we sit and wait for the animals to come to us."

Even better, there were no distractions in the process— no noise, no artificial interruptions, no digital diversions. In other words, *everything mattered.* Every experience was significant and potentially useful; every sensation provided valuable understandings of the world. Quality repetitions, powered by attention, powered by curiosity, powered by hunger, reinforced by occasional success. The process worked.

This pattern persisted for hundreds of generations, but then, as the media critic Neil Postman put it, "Change changed." As hunting and gathering gave way to agriculture, literacy, and numeracy, a new educational model began to take shape and little by little, we began to sit down and work at our desks. We spent less time studying habitat and more time working with symbols. For the first time in our history, we became literate, numerate animals.

NEW SCHOOL

As we understand it today, the Big Bang of modern education began with the work of the Greek philosopher and polymath Aristotle (384–322 BCE). His writings covered a broad range of subjects, including the natural sciences, philosophy, linguistics, economics, politics, psychology, and the arts. The breadth and depth of his knowledge was highly respected and was held as the essential touchstone for the educated person.

In fact, deep into the Middle Ages, the entire educational enterprise of the Western world consisted of little more than replicating Aristotelian knowledge, and in the world of medicine, Galen (129–199). A person (always a man) who mastered Aristotle or Galen's teachings would be granted a professorship. In turn, this became the model for the lecture-based classroom training that endures to this day. Sit still, listen to the professor, absorb and memorize what he has to say, then replicate it as accurately as possible. Modern schools around the world follow the same model. We've all been there.

All of which made a certain kind of sense in its day.

After all, Aristotle and Galen were respected tribal elders, and as humans, we naturally seek to learn from those who have gone before us. But the lecture-based model was historically abnormal and not exactly friendly to the human body. Even worse, it fundamentally shifted human attention away from the living, breathing world, toward abstract, symbolic representations. There was power in this process, of course, but displacement as well. For every hour we spend working with letters and numbers, that's an hour that we *don't* spend experiencing plants, animals, habitat, weather, and the night sky.

This radical diversion of human attention intensified with the work of René Descartes (1596–1650). Famous for his promotion of mind-body dualism, Descartes supposed that the mind was an independent entity, separate from and superior to the lower-order muscles, tissues, and organs of the body. Intelligence was all in the head, and thus, education must be symbolic, abstract, and lecture based. In the process, Descartes dealt a death blow to experiential education and left us with an archaic and often deadening neck-up, mind-over-body legacy that utterly fails to address the whole human animal in context.

In the modern classroom, education is still heavily influenced by the Aristotelian and Cartesian models, and has largely failed to accept, much less adopt, our modern understanding of neuroscience and the pivotal role of the body in the learning process. Within the neuroscientific community, embodied cognition is now universally recognized as fact, and we know full well that intelligence is broadly distributed across the entire body, not just the brain. And yet, modern education remains mired in a frustrating, confusing, and often counterproductive quagmire of competing ideas and practices.

Even worse, our educational systems are being crushed by the ever-growing complexity and acceleration of the modern world. As human knowledge has expanded, schools are now expected to teach all subjects and to solve social problems as well; we expect education to be all things to all people.

In the process, demands on students have escalated and created a toxic brew of stress, incessant work, and cognitive overload. Teachers are woefully underpaid and under extreme pressure to manage an increasingly unwieldly process. It's no surprise to see teachers quitting in droves and young people show almost no interest in joining the profession.

It's no wonder. Across all of modern education, from kindergarten to the highest ranks of academia, there is no truly unifying narrative about the purpose of the enterprise. We have no cultural *ikigai*, no coherent sense of meaning and purpose. In other words, we'd be hard pressed to even agree on what modern education is actually *for*. Is the purpose to perpetuate the dominant culture? Or is it to empower students? Is it for enlightenment? Or employment? Is it aspirational or utilitarian?

And without a unifying narrative, modern education often comes across as little more than just a monstrous pile of information to be scanned, processed, and sorted. In other words, it's incoherent.

All of which calls us to create a new-old model, something that's consistent not just with our history as hunters and gatherers but with modern discoveries in neuroscience. The good news is that the fundamentals are surprisingly easy to understand. We know the cellular basis of learning and the power of neuroplasticity. We know that the brain is a highly dynamic organ and that changes in synapses, neurons, and entire brain regions are almost always "use dependent." In short, repetitive experience is the primary driver of physical and mental transformation; reps are what make us who we are.

This new understanding may sound like a modern "discovery," and in some ways it is. But it's also consistent with the knowledge and teachings of our ancestors. Across a broad range of disciplines, from hunting and gathering to early literacy, to music, arts and crafts of a thousand varieties, our elders have always known that repetition is the key and that deep practice is the only thing that really works. In short, if we want to develop skill, we've got to put in the time and especially, the effort. Taken together, this shared understanding of human learning could be, or should be, the basis of human education and experiential design going forward.

WIRE TOGETHER

As it stands, many of us in the modern world are becoming fluent in the language of the nervous system, including a basic understanding of neurons, synapses, brain regions, and neural networks. Even in popular conversation, we hear people talking about the vagus nerve and its role in therapy, or the enhanced activity of the amygdala in trauma. People even use neurological metaphors in casual speech, as in "I'm carving a new groove in my nervous system."

But this was not always the case. In fact, as recently as the early days of the twentieth century, people didn't even understand the basic structure of the nervous system.

We knew nothing about neurons and we argued about whether the nervous system was one thing or many things. It seems incredible today, but it actually took an immense amount of dedicated effort to isolate the synaptic junctions between nerve cells and to recognize their role in learning and behavior.

The giant in this field was Santiago Ramón y Cajal, a winner of the Nobel Prize in 1906 for his work in describing the structure of the nervous system. His description of the synapse laid the groundwork for later discoveries through the rest of the century. Without this understanding of the synapse and the structure of neurons, there would be no neuroscience as we know it today.

Obviously, Ramón y Cajal was a clever scientist and a pathfinder in his era, but he got one thing dreadfully wrong. In his early examination of brains and nerves, he saw a system that appeared—to his eyes—to be fundamentally static in nature. Limited by the techniques of his day, he was unable to see microscopic changes to membranes, synapses, or relationships between cells, much less the birth of entirely new cells to replace existing neurons.

He summarized his view of a static nervous system this way: "In the adult, the nerve paths are something fixed and immutable.... Everything may die, nothing may be regenerated."

This orientation, later described as *neurofatalism*, became a widely accepted dogma both within and outside the neuroscientific community. For most of the twentieth century, students were taught that the nervous system simply doesn't change over time. In fact, it doesn't really do much besides fulfill its primary, inborn function; all it really does is carry messages from one place to another.

There's no growth, no significant learning, and no transformation. When it comes to brain cells, what you've got is what you're born with; nerve cells can only die.

This narrative was extremely influential across society at large, especially in the domains of education, management, and even athletic training. In essence, it told a story of innate traits, skills, and capabilities. People were either gifted or not. Students and athletes were born with particular inclinations and the only real challenge was to pigeonhole them into the right disciplines, arts, or sports. If we could put people into the right programs, they would flourish, but otherwise, they could only become slightly better versions of what they already were. There could be no major transformations, no success in alternate careers, no real creativity. Thus the label "fatalism."

This narrative held sway for most of the twentieth century and drove entire industries in intelligence and aptitude testing. Children and young athletes were rigorously assessed, measured, and evaluated for preexisting talents. Education was simply a matter of getting the evaluation right, at which point everything else would follow along in strict order, in theory at least.

But cracks began to show in the late 1960s with scientific discoveries revealing the dynamism of the nervous system. Little by little, we began to realize that every element in the system, from synapses to myelin sheaths to the cortex of the brain itself, was always in motion, always remodeling itself in response to the way it was used. Far from being a static structure, the nervous system was constantly transforming itself from minute to minute, hour to hour, and day to day.

This was a breathtaking and humbling insight. Suddenly,

we came to understand that the fatalistic dogma of the twentieth century wasn't just wrong, it was a massive distraction and a colossal waste of human and social potential. We were wrong about the brain and, in turn, we were wrong about learning, education, training, and even the nature of the human animal itself.

THE PROMISE OF NEURO-OPTIMISM

Fortunately, a new paradigm of neuro-optimism emerged with a far more promising narrative. Looking closer at the anatomy and electrochemical activity of synapses and neurons, scientists began to realize that when it comes to learning, almost anything is possible. Humans are wired for outrageous feats of learning that go far beyond our presumed limitations. Keep practicing, keep training, and the skills will come. It's all about the reps.

The prime example of neuroplastic transformation is long-term potentiation, or LTP. This is the process by which synaptic membranes become increasingly receptive to messages from upstream neurons, all of which is driven by use. In short, the more an upstream neuron talks to its downstream counterpart, the more efficient the communication becomes.

All of which might not sound like much. After all, synapses are microscopically small and this might even sound like an obscure bit of neuro wonkishness. But when we realize that this process of adaptation takes place constantly across billions of synapses in the brain and nervous system at large, we begin to get the picture. That is, the system is in constant motion, continually revising itself in response to repetitive experience. In this sense, learning never really sleeps. We're always in the act of remodeling ourselves in anticipation of future experience.

Looking at the big picture of human evolution and ancestry, this all makes perfect sense. When we're born into the world, we have no idea what kind of challenges we'll encounter. We might have to run or walk long distances; we might have to climb trees, chip stone tools, or today, deal with the overwhelming complexity of the modern world. All the body can really do is experience, observe, and feel, waiting for the reps to reveal the nature of its world and what the future might hold.

All of which yields another surprise. In popular culture, we hear a good deal about "the wisdom of the body," but in another sense, this is hardly the case. In fact, our understanding of neuroplasticity tells us that the body is essentially reactive. As complex and amazing as it is, physiology doesn't have the foresight to predict what's coming.

Instead, the body lies in wait for experience to tell it how to manage its resources and remodel itself. We might even go so far as to say that the body is rather dumb, but this "dumb like a fox" is actually a fantastic evolutionary strategy for living in an ambiguous and sometimes dangerous world. When you don't know what the future holds, it's a good idea to listen for repetitive patterns and remodel your tissue accordingly. If you can feel the rhythms of experience, you can build a functional body that will survive.

Neuroplasticity is all the rage these days and for good reason. It gives us the enormously optimistic lesson that, in theory at least, we can learn almost anything. It's a great message, but the potential goes even further than the motor skills we develop in sports, music, or art. In fact, a substantial body of work suggests that neuroplastic transformation takes place even with the most subtle qualities of the human experience, things like emotion, cognition, attitude, and judgment.

In other words, when it comes to human capability, it's all muscle. Everything we feel, say, or do is potentially trainable. We become better at love, anger, hurrying, compassion, or creativity precisely by practicing these very things. We get more courageous by exercising courage. We get better at slowing down by slowing down. We get better at persisting with difficult tasks by persisting in difficult tasks. We become more resilient by practicing resilience. We get better at paying attention to our breath by paying attention to our breath. Even our humanity itself is muscular; we either use it or lose it. In other words, it's all skill, all the way down.

All of which is inspiring but also sobering. In days gone by, we were conditioned to believe that the more subtle skills and qualities of our experience were simply given to us at birth; things like emotion and character were nothing more than fixed aspects of our personality. From this perspective, we believed that people were intrinsically angry, compassionate, patient, curious, calm, or nurturing. But now we know better; in essence, nothing about us is permanent and, in a very real sense, everything we feel, think, and do can be developed. All we have to do is put in the time and the effort.

We also come to the astonishing realization that every moment of our lives is a rep. In other words, we're always practicing something. Whatever you're doing right now is your practice. If you want a particular quality or skill for yourself, start practicing that quality. If you want a particular quality for your students, clients, or athletes, guide them in training for that particular thing. In theory at least, it's simple.

But the benefits of neuroplasticity go even further. It's easy to see how practiced repetition builds motor skill and even the more nuanced qualities of our personalities and our relationships with the world. But there seems to be a general benefit for the whole animal as well. By practicing consistently and making progressive gains in skill development, we lead the whole animal into integration and, in turn, a greater overall sense of confidence and comfort in the world at large. And the details don't seem to matter much. Reaching for mastery in *any* art or discipline has payoffs that extend beyond the cluster of neurons in question. The human animal thrives on progressive challenge, whatever form it might take.

To be sure, neuroplasticity and quality reps aren't going to overcome every obstacle, hardship, or limitation. We all have our own personal advantages and disadvantages, genetic gifts and deficits. Everyone has a history and culture that shapes their bodies and brains in particular ways. And, yes, if you're starting late in life, you probably aren't going to win the Tour de France or put up a new route on Mount Everest.

Likewise, if your community or culture fails to support your ambition, it's going to be an uphill struggle. Not everyone has a clear path to success; not everyone has the physical or social resources it takes to achieve mastery. It's also true that hard work sometimes fails and we might have to change course in our training and aspirations. Your chosen path might turn out to be a step in the wrong direction and might have to backtrack or switch paths entirely.

Nevertheless, neuroplasticity remains an immensely

powerful, underrated capability that we can harness to do incredible things. No matter our intrinsic gifts or limitations, our potential is vast. Adversities and limitations are real, but the human animal is far more capable than most of us realize. Human history is marked by struggle, but it also tells a story of ordinary people who have persisted in the face of overwhelming odds and succeeded beyond all expectation.

As coaches, teachers, and therapists, we always want to meet people where they are and avoid peddling fantasy. Nevertheless, our focus must always be on the horizon of possibility. Honor your people's history, circumstances, and limitations, but keep your eye on their potential. This is where the real action is.

EXECUTION

Neuroplasticity and neuro-optimism are exciting and practically useful concepts. Not only do they tell us how we learn, they also open our imagination to the idea that given enough effort, dedication, and practice, the human animal can learn incredible things.

The really good news is that we know just how to do it. In essence, neuroplastic transformation is all about quality reps, attention, and precision. We become what we focus on; we become what we repeatedly do. Studies of high performers in multiple domains, especially athletics, all point to the same conclusion. That is, skill development is the result of committed engagement, sometimes described as "deep practice" or "deliberate practice."

There's no secret to any of this. People who achieve high levels of mastery do so because they put in the time in highly focused efforts. Some may be blessed with ideal musculature or highly responsive nervous systems, but the main event will always be deep concentration in practice. There are no shortcuts.

Of course, our ancestors knew all this a long time ago. The Zen master Shunryu Suzuki put it this way:

> When you do something, you should do it with your whole body and mind; you should be concentrated on what you do. You should do it completely, like a good bonfire. You should not be a smoky fire. You should burn yourself completely.

And it's not just Zen masters. It's safe to assume that the cave painters of the Paleolithic, the great artists of the Renaissance, and every other high performer in history has understood the same basic principle: If you want to develop a skill or an aptitude, you've got to put in the time and the concentration.

It all makes perfect sense, but it also stands in sharp contrast to modern convenience culture and our prevailing practice of shallow engagement and dabbling. As traditional practices have eroded, so too has our ability to concentrate and learn. We've lost our respect for process; today we feel free to drop in and drop out of learning environments at will. We show up late, leave early, and even when we're physically present, we're often distracted by everything else that's going on in our lives. This adds up to poor-quality reps, wasted effort, and bad outcomes. And, as Arnold Schwarzenegger famously put it, "Garbage reps give garbage results."

This understanding forces us to confront modern culture head-on, especially what we might call "the war on

Zen," the combination of social forces, processes, and technologies that fragment our awareness and cripple our capacity for intelligent action. Sadly, this is the world we're living in: intrusive marketing and advertising, constantly selling fantasy, products, and memes that distract us from essential, core experiences.

Not only do our devices interrupt us throughout the day, they also grease the skids between stimulus and response, creating a "frictionless experience" that encourages us to act on every fleeting impulse. This kind of experience degrades human learning and function, fragments our consciousness, distorts and obscures reality, and erodes our freedom. Ultimately, distraction culture doesn't just cripple our neuroplastic potential, it also degrades our intelligence, our creativity, and our ability to build a functional future.

START SLOW

Ultimately, deep, focused practice is the name of the game. No matter the domain, our challenge is to bring the totality of the human animal to bear on the selected task. It doesn't matter whether we're lifting weights or writing an essay. It doesn't matter whether we're practicing guitar chords or learning how to fly an airplane. When it comes to concentration, more is more. Look for complete immersion and sustained focus for as long as possible; maximal attention to the matter at hand is what works. To personalize it, we might say, "I'm going to my entire being to this task in this moment." Even if you're feeling distracted or fragmented by other events in your life, you can still bring everything you've got.

But pace is also important. As we dive into our training,

our enthusiasm and passion for results can sometimes give us an exaggerated sense of urgency. We want our people to succeed, so we push the pace and leap ahead to more advanced material. Bored by the fundamentals, we try to accelerate the process and reach our destinations as fast as possible. But this rush to skill can compromise our efforts and even take us in the wrong direction entirely.

Instead, remember the classic metaphor for neuroplastic transformation: a drop of water falling on a hilltop. The earliest drops carve a shallow groove, but they also set a course for the drops that come later, eventually creating a deeper groove, then a rut, a gully, a stream, a valley, then finally, a canyon. If the early watercourse goes in the right direction, all will be well and the skill in question will be functional, athletic, and graceful. But if things go astray at the outset, it'll take heroic efforts to readjust the flow at some later date.

Novelist Paulo Coelho recognized the power in this process and emphasized the importance of early attention and care. As he put it, "Go slowly at the beginning, because direction is more important than speed." He was speaking as a writer, but his observation is spot on for any sort of skill development in any domain. Charging ahead toward some vague idea of mastery is folly; going fast in the wrong direction only gets us further away from what we're trying to do. Instead, start with discipline and clear objectives. Go slow, take your time, work with a teacher or coach, and get it right at the earliest moment. Or, if you're the leader, keep your students, clients, and athletes on track. Early precision is the key to success.

MUSIC GETS IT RIGHT

No matter the details of our practices and training objectives, all of us can also take inspiration from the world of musical training. As it turns out, music teachers follow an ideal pattern for neuroplastic transformation in the way they structure their lessons.

Variations abound but in general, the typical music lesson begins with some kind of tune-up and warm-up. Nothing fancy, just a transition from regular life to focused concentration on the instrument and the music. Next comes a few disciplined drills—scales, chords, and rhythmic fundamentals—to build foundational skills. Then, a review of familiar pieces, looking for more intense concentration and quality reps.

Then, a climax of sorts. As the student enters the sweet spot of stress and is primed for maximum learning, the teacher introduces some new and more challenging material. This is the heart of the lesson; as the student grapples with the difficulties, he brings everything he's got to the piece in question. The teacher sustains this phase as long as possible, until the play begins to sound sloppy, awkward, or forced.

Finally, the lesson concludes with a period of play and improv, looking to integrate the fruits of the discipline into an unconscious, effortless effort. Repeat this process a few thousand times and you've got a musician.

PRECISION STRESS

As we've seen, skill development is all about quality reps, attention and concentration, but getting the stress right is essential to everything we're trying to do. The good news is that we have a clear understanding of the neurobiology and how it works in training and practice. That is, when it comes to learning and memory, stress is a frenemy.

Like most things in the human body and in natural systems in general, the effect follows an inverse U-curve of benefit. At small doses and in moderation, stress hormones enhance the process of long-term potentiation at the synapse and solidify memories in certain brain regions, especially the hippocampus. At this level, stress is a powerful partner in skill development. If you're a teacher, trainer, coach, or parent, you very much want your people to be under a moderate, optimal level of stress when training and practicing.

But of course, the inverse U-curve tells us that there's bound to be a tipping point, a zone of diminishing returns, and in the worst case, a complete reversal of the learning process. When we pump too much cortisol into the nervous system, learning and memory begin to deteriorate and may collapse entirely. Even worse, the very same hormones have an opposite effect in the brain region dedicated to fear and surveillance: the amygdala. In other words, as stress escalates we become increasingly vigilant and focused on survival, just as we become less capable of learning and memory. Obviously, this is not the result we're looking for.

In popular culture, there's a growing understanding and appreciation for the negative effects of stress, but the standard narrative often suggests that our goal should be to eradicate stress entirely. In fact, advertisers often tell us that our lives can and should be stress-free. But this interpretation is both misleading and counterproductive. In fact, our goal should be proportion and precision, not eradication. We want to keep our people in the sweet spot of stress while they perform their high-quality reps. Think of it as a Goldilocks zone of experiential design; we're looking for just the right level of stress hormones in our students and athletes; go too far in either direction and you're going to have problems.

But how do we find that sweet spot? Naturally, there's huge individual variation here and conditions are always changing. Everyone has their own personal stress history, personal tolerance, and preference. For both individuals and groups, an optimal stress level today might be wildly inappropriate tomorrow. As Heraclitus would have put it, "You can't step into the same sweet spot twice." People's appetite for stress changes by the day and even by the hour.

Some trainers suggest that we can track stress levels with sophisticated devices that measure cortisol levels and while this might have some promise, it distracts us from more fundamental human skills, especially listening and simple observation. Knowing a particular data point about an athlete's stress hormone level doesn't really tell us that much anyway. What we really want to know are trends and the person's overall state of function.

HONOR THE TIPPING POINT

All of which suggests that we pay more attention to the overall disposition and non-verbal signals coming from our students, clients, and athletes. Changes in a person's stress status may come well before they're aware of it and may be reflected in their posture, tone of voice, facial expressions, and overall demeanor, especially their sense of humor. This will help us recognize patterns in their stress experience and, in particular, the point of diminishing returns.

As stress increases and your people approach the top of the curve, be alert for these warning signs:

- Anhedonia, or loss of pleasure, especially in activities that were formerly pleasurable

- Neophobia, the avoidance of new experiences, a diminished sense of adventure

- Increased reliance on familiar patterns of movement, behavior, and thought

- Reduced ambiguity tolerance, inability to deal with change and complexity

- Social withdrawal and isolation

- Cognitive distortions, especially overgeneralizing and black-and-white thinking

- Physical lethargy, poor sleep quality, decreased resilience, increased pain sensitivity

- General irritability and short temper, otherizing people and the world in general

- Catastrophizing, going straight to the worst-case scenario (making mountains out of molehills)

- Grim demeanor, especially decreased sense of humor and play

- Poor concentration and reduced attention span

- Impulsive behaviors and reduced self-control

- Decision resistance, procrastination, and impatience

EXPLANATORY STYLES

These behaviors and qualities are dead giveaways for hyper-stress, but you'll also want to pay close attention to the stories that people tell about themselves and their experience in the world; in short, we listen for their explanatory style. Work by psychologist Martin Seligman suggests that people on the verge of hyper-stress, depression, and learned helplessness interpret events in a way that's personal ("I suck."), pervasive, ("I suck at everything.") and permanent ("I'll always suck."). If you hear variations on these themes, listen closer; it may be time to make an adjustment.

Research also suggests that there's a significant physiological difference between stressors that are perceived as a challenge and those that are perceived as a threat. Work by June Gruber at Yale showed that stressors perceived to be challenging had beneficial physical effects, including increased strength of heart contractions, increased cardiac output, increased diameter of circulatory vessels, increased blood flow to the brain and muscles, and increased cognitive and physical performance. But when the stress is experienced as a threat, everything goes the other way, into a state of psychophysical contraction and reduced performance.

All of which may be reflected in a person's language. Do your students or athletes sound confident or intimidated? How do they describe their experience? Are they anticipating a meaningful, challenging struggle, or are they preparing for impending doom? Are they up for the task or are they overwhelmed? Listen closely and adjust accordingly. Their stories will tell the story.

FREEDOM AND DISCIPLINE

If we look at learning strictly in technical terms, the entire enterprise looks like a simple matter of getting the reps right. Quality practice, just inside the sweet spot of stress, will give us the results that we're looking for, and in theory, we could reduce the entire process to a rote set of guidelines, a template of reps or a spreadsheet of progressive tasks to be performed. In theory, we could just set the process in motion and let it run itself.

But people are more than just their brains, and more than just a bunch of fancy wiring. There's also the matter of personal history, imagination, and emotion. Does the experience feel playful and engaging, or does it feel onerous, limiting, or tyrannical? This brings up a crucial question: As coaches and teachers, should we encourage free, uninhibited practice, or should we hold our students' feet to the fire and demand perfection at every point in the process?

This is where we can find some clarity in the work of philosopher and mathematician Alfred North Whitehead and his book *The Aims of Education*, particularly his essay, "The Rhythmic Claims of Freedom and Discipline."

In Whitehead's day, a fierce debate raged in the educational community about the relative merits of rigorous discipline and free play, but Whitehead would have none of it. Instead, he took a big-picture view that embraced the benefits of both approaches. Advocating for a dynamic, natural approach that sounds almost Taoist, he called for a rhythmic, experiential oscillation: "Freedom and discipline are not antagonists, but should be so adjusted in the child's life that they correspond to a natural sway, to and fro, of the developing personality..."

For Whitehead, the ideal educational method—for adults and children alike—is best divided into two distinct phases: precision and romance. As we've seen, the precision phase is essential for forming functional pathways in the nervous system: getting the right cells to wire together into skillful, functional combinations. If we want to perform at a high level, our reps have to be as close to perfect as we can make them. For Whitehead, "This stage is dominated by the inescapable fact that there are right ways and wrong ways, and definite truths to be known." This is no time for improv, wanderlust, or playful interpretation; this is the time for focus.

But perfect reps only go so far, and for Whitehead, a playful romance phase was equally vital. As he saw it, "The organism will not absorb the fruits of the task unless its powers of apprehension are kept fresh by romance." In other words, there's got to be a psychological driver, a sense of potential, and a dream, if you will. If the athlete, student, or child has some sense of imagination and a vision of what might be possible, that person will persist, even in the face of hardship, confusion, and exhaustion.

This is where coaches, teachers, and parents can play a dual, ambidextrous role. It's almost as if you're two different people, alternating between two well-defined roles. When you're a precision coach, the job is all about discipline. You're going to be a strict task master. You'll demand the best from your people, with maximum focus and attention to detail. No matter how your people are doing, you're always there, encouraging them to do better.

In this phase, push for quality in execution and be assertive in correcting error. "Do it right, do it better, try it again." Mimic the music teacher: "Slow down, play those scales again, just so." Repeat until fatigue and sloppiness set in, then rest and do it again.

But when you're a romance coach, it's time for a completely different tone. Now it's all about the dream and the vision. It's all about painting a picture of what your people can become and how they'll feel along the way. Above all, it's a time to give meaning and purpose to what your people are aspiring to do. This is where the motivational talk comes in, this is where we speak in grand visions, of reaching the summit of whatever mountain your people might be climbing. This is where we feed the imagination with superpowers, mythic animals, legendary heroes, and the great feats of real-world performers. And in this phase, more is certainly better.

This alternation between precision and romance is an ideal pattern for education and training of all varieties, but it poses a big challenge for the aspiring coach, trainer, or leader. That is, most of us arrive in adulthood with something approaching a singular identity and, in a general sense, we know who we are. So we stake out a single position in our coaching style, with a tone and attitude that's consistent with our personality and our view of the world. Satisfied with who we are, we stick to it for years and even decades. In the process, our coaching style becomes one consistent, static, and maybe even lifeless thing.

But to succeed, we've got to be flexible in our identity and strive to master both styles of leadership; we've got to be capable of both precision *and* romance. In addition, we've got to be intentional about all of this, with distinct alternation between phases. A common rule of navigation in unfamiliar terrain tells us: "Know where you are at all times." But for our purposes it's: "Know *who* you are at all times." In this moment of training and practice, are you a precision coach or a romance coach? Get this straight in your mind and the process will go a lot easier for everyone.

HABIT REVISION

For anyone with an interest in becoming a more skillful and functional human, neuroplasticity is the most exciting game in town. We know how it works and, in one sense at least, it's pretty easy. Just put in lots of quality reps with lots of rest and the skills will come.

But it's not all good news for the learner because plasticity—for all its promise—also leads us into habits of behavior, sensation, and cognition that may or may not be adaptive.

In fact, plasticity and habit are inextricably related; they're two sides of the same process. In 1890, the psychologist William James observed that living creatures are nothing if not "bundles of habits." No matter who we are or how we live or train, habit is inevitable and unavoidable. Every time we do anything, we're facilitating neural pathways and, in the process, setting up habit patterns both large and small.

As trainers, coaches, teachers, and therapists, this is our beat, you might say. Recognize it or not, we're all in the habit business. We train the brain and the nervous system so that some skills and behaviors become faster and easier, while others are allowed to die out and become extinct. We give our people quality repetitions that help them adapt to their circumstances, to excel at sport, learning, and life; if we set this up properly, they'll go on to some kind of success.

COMPLICATIONS

But the challenge is more complex than we might imagine. Technically speaking, a habit is nothing more than a nervous system circuit that's been potentiated or facilitated by repetition. You've used a pattern repeatedly and now that circuit has wired together, and it might even feel like you're stuck with it.

But humans are more than electrochemical machines, and the nervous system is more than just a bunch of fancy wiring. Likewise, habits are more than just isolated, stand-alone circuits that trigger particular behaviors. That's because habits also have meaning and associations that go far beyond their immediate functionality.

Habits can serve larger purposes beyond the mere execution of a particular movement or behavior. They can even act like reinforcing scaffolding that holds our lives together, especially in the face of stress and ambiguity. Habits—even maladaptive habits—give our lives a comforting sense of coherence, certainty, and predictability, something to fall back on in the midst of chaos. We may not be able to predict or understand the chaos of the modern world, but we can at least depend on our morning and nightly routines. Which, of course, is why we cling to habits so fiercely. When our habits come to define and protect our identity and our way of life, we'll do everything we can to keep them in place.

And there's further complication that comes from our ferociously hypersocial nature. Like human brains, habits don't exist in isolation. Because our nervous systems are socially linked, our habits are continuously influenced by the people around us, either reinforced or discouraged by what everyone else is doing. In other words, habits come and go, not simply by way of our own personal willpower but also by virtue of what everyone around us is doing. If our peers are tweaking their habits in one direction or another, there's a good chance that we'll follow along.

Similarly, it also makes sense to talk about habit at larger scales. Call it tradition or cultural inertia if you will, there's a powerful tendency for cultures to persist with established customs, rituals, and ideas, even in the face of obvious dysfunction. This is particularly true in times of social stress and, now, ecological dysfunction. When human animals are under pressure, there's a powerful, unconscious inclination to revert to the familiar; when the going gets tough, we go back to what we know.

In this sense, there really is something to the notion that society develops habits and that those large-scale habits inevitably reflect back onto our personal behavior. We might like to think of ourselves as free agents, but there's no escaping the social world and the habits of mind and behavior that circulate through culture. And if those habits are deeply embedded in society, there's a good chance that they'll take us along for the ride.

THE ART OF UNLEARNING

In any case, the question on everyone's mind is: How do we edit, revise, or break our undesirable habits? Or to put it more specifically, How do we unlearn behaviors that no longer serve us? Surely there must be some magic formula, procedure, or mind-set that will liberate us from our various behavioral dysfunctions and maybe the experts can tell us what it is.

But we already know the fundamentals. Technically speaking, the entire challenge of habit revision should come down to quality reps, and in theory at least, we already understand how to do this. In fact, the formula for habit revision should be identical to our formula for establishing a habit in the first place. That is, we seek out quality reps in the new, adjusted direction. We apply as much attention as possible to the task at hand and try to let the older, undesirable habits fade away. This is precisely the method that musicians use to progress in their art; keep moving ahead toward new skills and let the awkward movements atrophy on their own time.

As for strategies for habit revision, opinions vary. Some coaches advocate the Japanese concept of *kaizen*: small changes pursued with diligence, especially a persistence fueled by some larger passion, an *ikigai*, a sense of meaning and purpose. It's a promising idea and it seems to be backed up by some real-world experience and research. Huge changes can fire up the stress-response system and sabotage the entire effort, but small changes are less threatening. It makes sense, but backsliding is a constant challenge. That's why coaching is so helpful; nudge your people toward the small changes and keep nagging until you get the transformation you're after.

But others advocate for bold, large-scale change; if we do something drastic with our lives, the new condition will overpower many of the habits in question. If you've ever traveled to a foreign country, particularly one with a completely different culture, you know how this works. Suddenly, you can't rely on your established habits of dress, money, food, language, or much of anything else. You've got to be intentional in all these things, and in the process, familiar habits tend to fade into the background.

Yet another approach is somatic and neurological. In

this practice, we look to prioritize the health and function of the brain's prefrontal cortex, that part of the brain that, in the words of Robert Sapolsky, "makes us do the harder thing." If the frontal cortex is weakened by chronic stress, alcohol addiction, or trauma, it won't fulfill its function of inhibiting impulse, and it's much more likely that we'll fall back into established habit patterns. The solution here lies in our familiar forms of relaxation therapy, social support, reduced workload, and contact with nature. Take care of the animal and the brain will do its job.

Likewise, we look to the art of slowing down, especially the Japanese concept of *yutori*, making space in our lives. This means turning down the pace and the workload, allowing more room for our humanity and our animal bodies to do what they need to do. This is where we can make room for deliberate intent. As Viktor Frankl put it, "Between stimulus and response there is a space. In that space is our power to choose our response…" In other words, if we can slow down, even a little, we'll be less likely to fall back into unconscious, automatic routine. We can choose.

All of which suggests yet another strategy, even a meta-strategy. In the popular imagination, we're likely to think of habit revision as something for occasional use, something we do when our lives go off the rails or some behavior becomes completely intolerable. If we succeed, we simply move on with our lives and forget the whole thing. To put it another way, we don't make a habit out of habit revision.

But habit revision can and should be treated as a foundational skill in itself. Thinking like athletic coaches once again, we realize that our training must always be specific to the outcome we're trying to achieve. In other words, if we want to become adept at revising habits, we've got to practice revising habits. So we apply ourselves to habit revision again, and again. Like musicians who constantly take on new pieces and new forms, we practice making and abandoning patterns, as a matter of course. In this practice, we learn to let go, to relinquish our attachment to familiar behaviors, and to live in some new way. We'll never become completely habit-free, nor would we want to be, but our habits will become a lot less tyrannical.

TRUST THE PROCESS

The problem with learning is that it usually takes a lot of reps to get what we're after. If you're young or lucky, you might be able to pick up a skill without much effort, but for the rest of us, there's got to be, as martial art teachers put it, "time on the mat." Not just hours or weeks of dabbling, but years of dedicated effort. We've all heard the claim that it takes 10,000 hours to develop mastery in anything, but whatever the actual number, it's sure to be a long time.

The problem is that humans are complicated animals, and putting in the reps isn't always a straightforward process. In fact, there are plenty of emotional, historical, and personal obstacles that can stand in our way. We want the skill, but the process feels daunting, effortful, and intimidating. We want to transcend where we are, but we're reluctant to go into the zone of discomfort. We want what the experience promises, but we're not sure we're ready to push ourselves so far.

The good news is that anxiety and frustration are actually signs that neuroplasticity is imminent; discomfort means that the brain is on the verge of transformation.

Neuroscientist Andrew Huberman explains how the process works:

> The agitation and stress that you feel at the beginning of something—when you're trying to lean into it and you can't focus: you feel agitated and your mind's jumping all over the place—that is just a gate. You have to pass through that gate to get to the focus component.

"Forget how you feel right now" he adds. It's going to feel good eventually, "but there's a whole staircase in which it feels kind of lousy.... The early stages of hard work and focus are always going to feel like agitation, stress, and confusion."

In other words, there's a sticking point right at the outset. If we can get past the point of discomfort and into the flow of practice, we've got a shot at some real plasticity and skill development. In turn, this is where things start to snowball as the process builds on itself.

The challenge is that practice can feel like drudgery, especially on bad days. You've got to apply conscious, deliberate attention to what you're doing and, worst of all, you don't have any skills to play with. It's just not much fun, and not surprisingly, many people simply quit at this point. Every music teacher in the world knows how this works: for every student who sticks with it, there's a hundred who drop out when the going gets tough.

But if we can get past the sticking point, things will start to get interesting. Once we get a few solid skills established, we can fire the imagination with a sense of possibility. New discoveries in movement and sensation put us into a positive feedback cycle, and having fun makes us want to play more. We've got our teeth into it now and we can feel the energy that comes with a budding sense of mastery, or at least competence. When we really feel it, we actually begin to crave our practice sessions, and when this happens, there's nothing that can stop us.

TAKE A CHANCE

So this is the paradox of training; to develop new skills, we've got to go into the zone of discomfort, or as some have put it, "We've got to get comfortable with being uncomfortable." But of course, we resist and procrastinate. We cling to what's familiar, especially our physical comfort and our sense of control and predictability. Above all, we want to be safe.

But in the extreme, it's precisely this sense of safetyism that holds us back. In *The Coddling of the American Mind*, authors Greg Lukianoff and Jonathan Haidt define safety-ism as a culture or belief system in which safety is held as a sacred value and risk is something to be avoided whenever possible.

But like all things in the human experience, safety and comfort follow the classic inverse U-curve that we see in so many domains. A little bit is a good thing, a little more is even better, but sooner or later there comes a tipping point and a descent into diminishing returns and even toxicity. When our lives become too safe and comfortable, we lose contact with mystery and adventure. Life becomes shallow and deadening; we lose our vitality and exuberance, even our sense of life itself. In the extreme, safety kills the very thing it was meant to protect.

The antidote is to replace our reluctance and safetyism with a sense of adventure and a willingness to go toward discomfort. Of course you have doubts. You *should* have doubts about your ability, your skills, and your journey into the discomfort zone. If you didn't have doubts, there wouldn't be much point in doing it.

The problem is that it's not easy to feel our progress from day to day. We play the scales and chords over and over, we do the drills on the athletic field, we write long passages, and we sleep as deeply as we can. But on some days, it all feels like nothing is changing; we're still the same person as yesterday.

But things *are* changing. Neuroplasticity is always in motion. You're putting in the reps and the body knows it. You've stimulated microscopic changes across millions and even billions of synapses, myelin sheath wrappings are becoming tighter for faster transmission of nerve impulses, and your brain's sensory-motor cortex is rearranging itself. Rest assured, your body is getting the message. So too for your students, athletes, clients, and children. It may not be readily apparent, but a transformation is underway.

START HUNGRY, STAY HUNGRY

Neuroscience gives us a great instruction in the details of neuroplastic wiring and the power of repetition, but it doesn't tell us much about the motivation behind the process. Why do some people persist in their practice while others give up? All the technical drills in the world aren't going to help people who aren't hungry.

And on the flip side, if people are truly hungry for the learning, they'll stay engaged in the training process, even in the face of confusion, incoherence, and adversity. Quality reps are essential, but desire is equally vital, maybe even more so. As almost every athletic coach in the world has put it at some point, "You've got to want it."

This is where you come in. As you plan your experiential design and execute your programs, look for ways to keep the hunger alive. Keep looking for new ways to fall in love with the process. Tell stories of hungry people who've persisted in the face of adversity. Point out nuance in the training process, new sensations and experiences that people can feel and learn to appreciate. And above all, model your own hunger for continued learning. You may or may not be a master of the skill in question, but it's your love of the learning process itself that will keep people in the game. Ultimately, your hunger will be contagious.

CARROTS AND STICKS

For coaches, teachers, trainers, and parents, there's one final issue that relates to the matter of human learning and that's the matter of rewards and punishments. Some of us are apt to wonder: Can we improve the performance of our students, athletes, and children by offering them rewards for trying harder? Can we discourage them from bad behavior with punishments? If we offer the right carrots and sticks, people's behavior and performance should improve—so our reasoning goes.

These approaches and assumptions are extremely popular, but they also beg some obvious questions. Do rewards and punishments actually *work*? Do people learn better when bribed with carrots or punished with sticks? Should this be part of our experiential design?

A lot of people seem to think so. In fact, we see incentives all over modern society: classrooms, athletic fields, workplaces, shopping centers, banks, and commerce at large. As a society, we've come to believe that this kind of behavior modification works as intended, but what if we're wrong about all of this? And even more to the point, what if it succeeds in one way but creates something extremely destructive in the process?

The clearest answer to these questions comes from Alfie Kohn and his classic *Punished by Rewards: The Trouble with Gold Stars, Incentive Plans, A's, Praise, and Other Bribes*. As Kohn sees it, modern education and commercial society can now be boiled down to one simple stimulus-response prescription for behavior: "Do this and you'll get that." In other words, if you behave in a particular way, you'll get an external reward, independent of the original activity. Do this worksheet, play these chords and scales, do these reps, fill out this spreadsheet, purchase this product, and we'll give you a perk.

All of which might seem innocent enough, but in the process, the very nature of the game changes. The original act is devalued and becomes nothing more than an incremental step on the way toward getting the reward in question; beyond securing the perk, the activity has no particular value in and of itself. Instead, the reward becomes the prime objective while the means becomes irrelevant. Kohn summed up the research in human motivation this way: "The more we reward someone for doing something, the less interest they have in that thing."

Kohn is a classroom educator, but his observations apply equally across all domains of modern human experience. Rewards are all around us now, in our schools, our sports, and our careers. Taken together, this widespread practice leads many of us into unconscious and habitual behaviors. Constantly chasing rewards, we lose track of who we are and what we really want to do in the world.

This is the dark side of carrots and sticks; little by little, reward by reward, we lose our precious sense of meaning and purpose. This is a catastrophe not just for our ability to learn but also for our sense of wildness; the more we chase rewards, the more machine-like we become. Even worse, it's a self-perpetuating system. As Kohn put it, "Do rewards motivate people? Absolutely. They motivate people to seek rewards."

The antidote is to keep our focus on intrinsic rewards: the pleasure and satisfaction that comes with the original act, the original quest, the original discipline, whatever it might be. Keep as close as possible to your selected practice. Stay focused on the parts of the experience that are self-rewarding. Keep people's attention on intrinsic values and avoid external rewards whenever possible.

Naturally, people will push back against all of this. We've been conditioned to believe that dedicated practice is unpleasant work and that we need to reward people to keep them on task. But this is a fallacy—a myth that reflects our lack of imagination. In fact, the rewards are right there in the process; we just have to get better at seeing them, feeling them, and pointing them out to our students, clients, and athletes. To be sure, quality reps are demanding—they're supposed to be demanding—but progressive mastery also feels fantastic and motivating. Being challenged and getting better at anything is fundamentally satisfying. This is where our focus must be.

CHAPTER 6
MODELS

As we dig deeper into our experiential design for the human animal, we can take inspiration and guidance from a wide range of cultures, training, and educational practices. We wonder... How do humans learn? What kinds of settings and experiences move people to higher levels of function and equipoise? What kinds of teaching and coaching strategies seem to work best? How can we create magic with our students, athletes, and clients? By becoming students of learning itself, we refine our existing programs and methods or create entirely new ones from scratch.

There are many models to choose from, and we could borrow from almost any region of the world. Humans are adept at creating culture and, in particular, creating practices that move individuals and communities toward higher levels of function, health, and integration. We could spend years examining and taking inspiration from the various forms of practice that we find on every continent.

Nevertheless, there are three notable models that stand out, each making a vital contribution to our experiential design process: athletic training, martial art, and West African drum and dance. By studying these models, you'll gain a greater sense of possibility for your own creation.

Of course, you might well feel unqualified to fill any of these roles or to exercise leadership in the details of these practices. Maybe you're not an athletic trainer or a coach. Maybe you have no experience in the martial arts or in West African drumming. Not many people do. But never fear, technical expertise is not the issue here. The idea is not to replicate any of these models with precision, although if you chose to do so, you won't go far wrong. Rather, the point is to observe successful paradigms and see what makes them work.

Ultimately, you'll want to design an experience based on your own capabilities, skills, and resources. You might create a hybrid or integrate some particularly promising ideas from one model or another, but ultimately, this will be your creation. To be sure, we always want to honor traditions and the teachings of our elders and to give credit to those who came before us, but there's nothing to say that you can't borrow and incorporate ideas along the way.

And remember, even if you don't have the desired skills or experience to teach a particular skill, you can always invite guest teachers and coaches to join the classes or workshops that you produce. As a creator, the possibilities are endless.

THE ATHLETIC TRAINING MODEL

Our first model comes from the world of sports and athletic training, a powerful, proven method for developing high-functioning humans. Athletic training is one of the most effective practices in the modern world, and arguably, sport is one of the few things in modern society that actually functions as intended.

The process is simple and we know just how it works:

The rhythmic challenge of athletic training, coupled with deep rest, leads to impressive adaptations in the human body. Not only do most participants become physically stronger, faster, and more agile, they also gain a powerful sense of mastery and control.

Even better, athletic training gives participants a robust sense of coherence. That is, the challenge is easy to understand; all you need to do is master some basic skills and you'll have a shot at winning, or at least playing the game. The sheer simplicity of the enterprise offers a seductive and promising alternative to life in our hypercomplex, chaotic world.

Sport also succeeds when it provides life lessons that go beyond the game itself. Athletes train with intense dedication in a single domain and can use that experience as a model for learning and living in other contexts. By itself, mastery in running long distances, throwing a ball, jumping over a bar, or climbing an artificial wall has almost nothing to do with real life in the modern world. But under the direction of a wise coach or teacher, athletic practice can become a paradigm for anything we might choose to do later in life: "I trained hard and excelled in my sport, so I can probably succeed in this new challenge."

In fact, the world of sport provides us with a powerful, easily understood metaphor for living in the world at large. Inspired by the physical power and grace of great athletes, we begin to look for similar qualities off the field, off the court, and outside the bounds of the game itself. When confronted by the inevitable dilemmas in life, we look for qualities of mind and body that are both strong and flexible, stable and fluid; think of this as "athletic equipoise"

THE DARK SIDE

There are ample reasons to love athletics, and we'd do well to keep this spirit alive for athletes and nonathletes alike. Nevertheless, sport doesn't always live up to its potential, and anyone who's involved in experiential design needs to know that there's a very real shadow side to the athletic enterprise.

The most obvious issue is our obsession with competition and winning above all else. In fact, modern sporting culture has evolved to favor the "short win" over almost every other consideration. Destinations—championships and victories—are often held as the ultimate goal, while journey and process are devalued.

This competitive fixation is particularly regrettable in the world of youth sports, where professionalization and early specialization often lead to injury and burnout. Even worse, the competitive structure is systematically exclusionary, intentionally designed to weed out lesser prospects in favor of promising champions. The method is great for spectators who are looking for something spectacular, but from a public health standpoint, it's sheer folly. Why should it be that only the elite players get to enjoy the benefits of sport? Why should lesser talents have to warm the bench? Isn't sport for everyone?

In fact, the competitive mindset can distract us from other, vitally important experiential objectives. Even more than winning, participants want the feeling that comes with play and mastery. We want to feel competent and skillful; we want the sensations that come when our bodies move with power, agility, and grace. To be sure, this kind of experience can coexist with the quest for victory, but there's danger here; when we focus exclusively on winning, we can lose touch with the exhilaration that comes with simply loving the game.

Worst of all, when the competitive value system comes to dominate, individual players effectively become disposable. This is most obvious in professional sports, but the attitude is becoming pervasive across society. People are now considered valuable only to the extent that they can provide a very narrow service to the team, the company, or the workforce. If they fail to perform in that service—if they're injured or slowed by the passage of time, they're quickly disposed of. This brutally exclusionary process can make for some spectacularly high-performing teams and athletic stars, but it's hell for everyone else.

THE POWER OF FUNCTION

Putting these reservations aside for the moment, it's clear that athletic training offers some powerful lessons we can apply in our work with students, clients, and even children. In particular, it's especially valuable in the way it focuses our attention on function, not appearance. The whole point of the sporting enterprise is to create effective athletic movements: throwing, catching, hitting, or shooting a ball, for example.

In all these cases, success is measured by an athlete's ability to do a particular set of movements extremely well, and it doesn't matter what she happens to look like in the process. If you can get the ball through the hoop or over the goal line, your coach is going to be happy.

This approach also aligns perfectly with the mission of physical therapy and rehabilitation practices. That is, your therapist really doesn't care what you look like; her primary concern is that her patients can perform the desired movements effectively and without pain. In fact, athletic coaches and physical therapists are united in their critique of bodybuilding and cosmetic culture. As they see it, our obsessive attention to appearance serves as a real distraction to more important matters. Yes, we all want to look good, but in our quest to create lives that actually work, function is paramount.

The beauty of this approach is that it's fundamentally integrative for the body as a whole. In the language of physical therapists, athletic trainers look for movements that are multi-joint and multi-plane. Instead of isolating a particular muscle, trainers look to spread the load across long kinetic chains, orchestrating and coordinating sensation and movement. In practice, we look to create a conversation between the body and environment in ways that mimic real-world conditions. Ultimately, it's about the nervous system, especially proprioception, the sensation of position and momentum of our limbs and joints. In other words, it's always about skill.

This functional approach is vital for sporting success and rehabilitation in the wake of injury, but it also serves as a model and a metaphor for any other educational enterprise and our lives overall. Can we perform the task in question? Can we exercise skill in movement? Can we execute the challenge with grace, power, ease, and equanimity? This orientation is powerful not just for life on the athletic field but for anything else we might want to do, especially as we head into an ambiguous and challenging near-term future. When the chaos hits the fan, our physical appearance isn't going to matter much. Our ability to get things done in a rapidly changing world is what will carry the day.

SPECIFICITY

Closely related to the functional approach is the athletic trainer's dedication to specific training. When trainers work with athletes, the focus is always on particular performance outcomes. Coaches know the kind of changes they want to see and they work doggedly to create exactly those changes. In this effort, trainers and coaches follow a simple guideline, encapsulated in the buzzword SAID: Specific Adaptation to Imposed Demands.

In short, this is how the body works: Whenever we encounter a physical challenge, especially one that repeats in a rhythmic pattern, the body begins modifying tissue and information flows to support future instances of that same kind of challenge. The process is incredibly precise in this regard, right down to the molecular level. The body detects a pattern of experience, anticipates a similar future, and prepares by turning genes on and off, building tissue, and changing patterns of neuromuscular circuitry. The more specific the adaptation, the greater the chances for survival and success.

All of which adds up to a simple general principle for athletic training or training of any kind: If you want to create a particular performance or educational outcome, you've got to pay close attention to what you're trying to achieve. If you try to train a swimmer with long-distance running, you're not going to get good results. If you try to train a guitar player with squats and dumbbells, he's not going to make much progress either.

To put it another way, general conditioning is not enough. Being tough or resilient is not enough. As a coach or teacher, you want your athletes, clients, and students to develop particular skills and skill sets. Once you identify your objectives, you're on your way to creating an effective training program.

Going further, the SAID principle applies, not just obvious physical elements like strength, endurance, and agility but more broadly to *any* human capability. As we've seen in our conversation about neuro-optimism, plasticity works even in the most subtle domains of human experience. In other words, we can train our capacity for almost anything, from memory and concentration to empathy, compassion, gratitude, courage, and curiosity.

But you can't train for a condition, challenge, or predicament if you don't know what it is. If you don't have a clear understanding of your target objective, it's going to be nearly impossible to devise appropriate training for students, clients, athletes, or children. And yet, this is precisely where modern educational practices so often fail. We aren't training people specifically for the demands that they're going to encounter in the near-term future. In fact, we've scarcely given any thought to the matter. Judging from appearances, we simply assume that the near-term future is going to be pretty much like the near-term past. This is wishful, even delusional thinking and a recipe for disaster. As we've seen, tomorrow simply isn't going to be like today.

Unfortunately, modern education mostly ignores the vital lessons that come from the world of athletic training. In particular, we violate the SAID principle when we expect one kind of practice and training to produce some other kind of result. Most obviously, we seem to expect that academic knowledge, specialization, and rote memorization will somehow translate into competence later in life. But the body just doesn't work that way. If you really want to move the needle of human function, you've got to have a laser focus on context and the task in question.

To put it another way, we are utterly failing to harness the wisdom of the athletic coaching community to prepare the human animal for the near-term future. If we brought our coaches on board, they'd have a very clear understanding of how to proceed: First, examine the nature of the near-term future and the specific challenges that your people are going to face. Describe these challenges in detail, with as much precision as you possibly can. Second, start training specifically for these challenges. And that's it. In a conceptual sense at least, it's easy.

So the obvious question: What will be the nature of our near-term future? What are the actual, specific challenges and demands that the human animal will face? What kind of tasks will we need to perform as we enter this precarious state of ambiguity and ecological collapse? What are the skills and aptitudes your students, athletes, and offspring will need to survive?

Obviously, this is one messy inquiry, and it's almost impossible to predict exactly how ecological challenges will impact any particular group of people. Nevertheless, we can say that in a general sense, the near-term future promises high levels of ambiguity, stress, and disorienting change. We're likely to see shortages of critical supplies, including food, water, medicine, and materials.

Likewise, we'll probably see increases in social stress, including shifting hierarchies and relationships that no longer function in expected ways. As supply chains break down and social services begin to fragment, people will need to grow more of their own food, take care of more of their own housing and transportation, handle more of their own medical care, and manage all of this in an atmosphere of increasing stress.

To narrow it further, we'd say that the near-term future calls for an increased emphasis on practical, physical, manual skills, coupled with psychological flexibility. We're going to need people who can use simple tools, make repairs, dig gardens, push wheelbarrows, work with a variety of materials, perform first-aid, and build community.

Even more to the point, we're going to have to improvise. Conditions are going to be suboptimal, and we simply aren't going to have the right tools, materials, or knowledge that we need. And in keeping with our athletic coaching model, all these challenges should be approached as trainable skills. In other words, we get good at improvising with what we've got on hand by doing exactly that: improvising with what we've got on hand.

PRECISION STRESS

Not only does athletic training show us the power of specificity and function, it also offers participants a highly concentrated experience of quality repetition and, in turn, a genuinely transformative learning experience. As we've seen, quality reps are built on precision, focused attention, and concentration, powered by a sense of meaning and dedicated effort. Coaches and trainers understand this better than almost anyone else in the modern world. When practice begins, they strip away distractions and drive their athlete's attention with simple instructions and clarity. They know the drill: Quality reps give quality results.

But it's not just the reps or the movements themselves. Athletic trainers and coaches also possess a keen understanding of stress and what it means for the training process. In particular, they understand that the beneficial effects of stress follow the classic inverse U-curve: a little bit is really good, a little more is even better, but there's always a tipping point and a zone of diminishing returns, wasted effort, and tissue damage.

This is why athletic trainers put enormous effort into mapping and planning the stress levels of their athletes with periodization: macrocycles, mesocycles, and microcycles of training. It's all about creating ideal rhythms of effort and rest; if you can get the oscillation right, you'll have a successful athlete.

Not surprisingly, coaches also pay close attention to athletes who are approaching the tipping point of the inverse U-curve. They push their athletes as hard as possible but then back off as soon as they see some sign that they're going too far. Naturally, this requires a judgment call and it's not always an easy one. Biomedical monitoring offers some promise, but it's not always clear that any particular physiological metric will tell the story.

This is why experienced trainers and coaches pay close attention to their athletes' overall demeanor and relationship to the experience. In particular, they listen carefully to the ways their athletes describe their lived experience in drills, reps, and practice. Does the experience feel playful or is it workish? If workish, does it feel promising? Does it feel like a challenge or a threat? Does it pull them into the deeper engagement? Does it leave them wanting more or does it feel punishing and exhausting? Is this "good pain" or "bad pain?" This kind of inquiry is absolutely vital, not just in the world of sport, but in any learning enterprise.

JOURNEYS INTO THE RED ZONE

Of course, it's almost impossible to draw bright lines on any of this. Technically speaking, the whole idea of working the stress curve is to keep people in the sweet spot of optimal challenge. This is where stress hormones do their magic, ramping up the long-term potentiation of synapses, myelination of nerve fibers, and promotion of memory. And from this perspective, conventional wisdom tells us to avoid the red zone altogether. Excessive stress threatens to degrade tissue and reverse hard-won gains in training; if we can keep people in the green, everything will work better.

But in the living human animal, there's more to this process than tissue, synapses, myelin sheaths, and hormones. As it turns out, occasional journeys into the red zone of overstress and overtraining can have enormous psychological benefits for anyone who's trying to learn and live in a challenging world.

Naturally, the experience is going to be intimidating, overwhelming, and maybe even painful. And while it's hard on the nervous system in the short term, the experience will prove immensely valuable as a driver of self-discovery and ultimately, confidence and resilience. Having gone into action in hostile circumstances, the human animal finds strength in prior success. "I've been into the red zone before and survived. I can do it again."

In this sense, going into the red zone of stress can actually be a vital part of training. Take your clients, students, and athletes past the point of comfortable stress on occasion and you'll get better results in the long run. Yes, there will be minor, short-term injuries to tissue and neural circuits, and recovery might take longer than you'd like. But tissues will heal, the body will put itself back together, and people will be even stronger than before.

This is precisely what we see in many high-intensity sports, professions, and disciplines, and it's particularly the case in extreme professions like mountain climbing and military training. When you're going into action in a dangerous, potentially lethal situation, it's good to have some adverse experience in your background. So don't be afraid of taking your students, athletes, and clients into the red zone. When they've battled the dragon before and survived, they'll feel confident that they can do it again.

TEAM SPIRIT

Another life lesson that comes with the athletic model lies in the power of team sport. Players and fans understand how exhilarating and transformative this can be, and it's no wonder that we're so attracted to team sporting events. Faced with the shared predicament of athletic competition, everyone involved is having roughly the same autonomic experience at the same time; everyone on the team and in the stands is pumping the same hormones and everyone is exercising a similar fight-flight response.

The excitement of the shared experience can be stimulating and even intoxicating, but this is far more than a hormonal side effect of team competition. This is a profound process of social-physiological alignment, something that we rarely see in other settings. By giving our teams a clear sense of shared predicament, we're actually manipulating the flow of information in their bodies and, in turn, the flow of their cognition and spirit. Aside from battlefield combat or other shared predicaments like alpine climbing, such group alignment is rare in the modern world. Even the greatest motivational speeches fail to have such a dramatic psychophysical effect.

Even more interesting is the fact that this experience of autonomic unity is actually the historical norm for our species. Exposed and vulnerable in a wild grassland habitat, with predators never far away, people clustered in tribal groups for protection. And in these groups, there was always some sense of unity in the face of shared danger. We all agreed on the fundamentals: lions and leopards are dangerous; hippos and rhinos are dangerous; wildfires, gravity, and fast water are dangerous. Without even trying, we agreed on all of this and in turn, consensus was relatively easy.

This experience lives on in the world of modern team sports, where we feel a near-perfect consensus on the nature of our team's predicament. Opposing teams represent a threat, and a symbolic danger to our survival. They have big, fast players and we feel intimidated by their skills. Everyone on the team and in the stands understands the situation and responds with similar neurobiology. For a precious moment, or perhaps a season, our brains and bodies are one.

All of which provides a clear message that's staring us in the face. If we want the larger human team to work together, we've got to come to agreement on the nature of our predicament. In other words, we've got to recognize what's truly dangerous. In turn, this calls for leadership and sober, scientific evaluation of modern threats. What's truly dangerous right now? This would be a good time to get our team on board with reminders of actual threats to human life. Stop obsessing over false tigers and focus instead on the real lions, tigers, and bears that threaten to bring us all down.

THE MARTIAL ART MODEL

> The ultimate goal of karate is not winning
> or losing, but perfection of the character
> of its participants.
>
> —Gichin Funakoshi

As we look to craft whole-person, radically human experiences for our students, clients, and athletes, a particularly vivid example of experiential design comes to us from the world of martial art. As we'll see, this is one of the most successful and, for many, one of the most influential forms of experiential education on the planet. There are powerful life lessons here and important takeaways for anyone who works with the human animal.

Unfortunately, there's also enormous diversity in this world and it's not always easy to sort out what's really going on. There are dozens of styles and offshoots, and a wide variety of cultural practices that define the various teachings. There's a plethora of teachers, schools, and objectives, not all of which are pointed in the same direction. Nevertheless, when practiced with sincerity and dedication, martial art serves as a powerful experience that transforms lives, builds community, and promotes health.

A perfect example comes from the practice of aikido, where a simple ritual perfectly captures the essence of respectful relationships and sincerity in training. At the beginning of each session, the teacher-sensei bows to the class and says "Onegai shimasu," in a strong, assertive voice. Students return the bow and repeat the greeting.

It's a polite request: "May I please train with you?" Or,

"Thank you for the gift I am about to receive." Or, "I hope our relationship will be fruitful." The message is an expression of generosity, gratitude, an open mind, and cooperation. All of which sets an ideal tone for vigorous practice and serves as a model for other forms of experiential design. You probably don't speak Japanese and you probably won't use this particular greeting in your training, but you can look for similar ways to build this kind of tone and theme into your programs.

A CULTURE OF SKILL

But before digging deeper, it helps to know some broad outlines of Eastern culture and traditions. In the popular imagination, we're quick think of Buddhism and an attitude of calm reflection and equanimity in the face of change. In particular, we're reminded of the Buddha's legendary observation that "all life is impermanent and therefore unsatisfactory," or the popular "All life is suffering." If we can relinquish our attachment to security and permanence, then we'll be free to live in the moment.

It's a powerful teaching, but there's another thread in the Eastern tradition that's often lost in popular conversations: the importance of skill in movement and living. The early works of Taoism are particularly notable in this respect, especially *The Tao te Ching* and the writings of Chuang Tzu, where references to skill development are woven throughout. The Taoists were fascinated by expertise, both in daily tasks and in more challenging combative encounters. In fact, it's really a mistake to describe early Taoism as a religion at all; the ancient texts sound more like instruction manuals for living than guides for worshiping a deity.

The beauty of Taoism is that it brings us a vivid description of skill and effortless living, a practice and way of being known as *wu wei*. In short, this is the ultimate aspirational objective for training and practice. As we perform our sets and reps over the course of months and years, our skills increase to the point where our movements become effortless. This is the art of "inaction" and "inexertion," the ideal expression of skill in martial art, sport, craft, or any other discipline.

To our Western ears, *wu wei* sounds mystical and esoteric; something impossibly nuanced and only accessible to ancient masters of the distant past. But in fact, it's actually a sophisticated description of a neurological process that's present in every human discipline and art. Even better, the progression is simple and, today, well understood.

汉
字

We begin with conscious, intentional, and methodical reps, usually under the direction of a master teacher. At this level, the action is cortical, workish, and disciplined; we're using focused, conscious intent to change sensory and motor patterns in the cortex of the brain. Perform one move at a time, correct for error, then repeat. Try again, and repeat the process for weeks, months, and years.

It's a laborious process but little by little, neural activity begins to shift. Sensory-motor pathways become stable and in turn, the action sinks lower, into the limbic, subcortical regions of the brain and ultimately, into the body. Effort fades away and we begin to express ourselves through movement. With further practice, things become increasingly effortless as we move into the domain of *wu wei*. Ideally, every sensory and movement practice will follow this progression.

The path to *wu wei* holds true across every discipline and art. In the yang or discipline phase, we try as hard as we can. We intensify our effort and look for high-quality, precision reps. But as we move to the yin phase of training, we look to execute will less and less effort. We're doing the same movements or tasks, but without trying. In the process, we get out of our heads and let our bodies take over. While the yang phase was all about effort and precision, the yin phase is all about ease, fluidity, and trust in the body.

The challenge is that most of us in the West have been trained exclusively in the active, yang phase of practice. Across modern culture, we're constantly encouraged to try and try harder. We prime ourselves with motivational speeches, motivational devices, and motivational chemicals. We urge one another to be more productive and we reward those who are relentless in their effort. In this kind of culture, the yin art seems strange, unfamiliar, and even just wrong. We're conditioned to try harder, but almost no one tells us to "try softer." Almost no one tells us to relinquish our striving and let our skills come forth.

The process of moving into *wu wei* is neurological but also hinges on our relationship with ourselves. That is, the ultimate expression of skill comes when we relinquish our self-consciousness and our self-image. The challenge is particularly acute for those of us who've trained hard to develop a set of capabilities. We've come to identify with a particular skill and in turn, we're quick to defend that identity. Error would be a threat to our self-image, so we redouble our effort and, in the process, our movements stiffen and become labored. We lose our sense of play.

Musicians know this paradox well; identification with high performance inhibits high performance. Author Kenny Werner puts it this way in *Effortless Mastery: Liberating the Master Musician Within* "Surrender is the key, and the first thing to surrender is one of your most prized possessions: your obsessive need to sound good." In other words, the more we identify with ability and mastery, the more we inhibit the flow of *wu wei*. "When you don't try as hard to be good, you play better... By not caring, you play better." Abandon your fear, your ego, and your quest for excellence. Just play. Or as Stephen Nachmanovitch put it in *Free Play: Improvisation in Life and Art*, "For art to appear, we have to disappear."

All of which suggests two very different styles of practice. In the first stage, we're all about quality reps, discipline, focused labor, and intensity. We practice our movements with as much precision as possible and drive the process forward with intention. Diligent and dedicated, we sustain this approach for months and years. But as our bodies begin to soak up the training and skill begins to run on its own, we adopt a different attitude and relationship to our practice. Now we trust the body to do what it knows how to do.

If you're a teacher, trainer, or coach, you'll want to

support this ambidextrous approach, depending on what state your people happen to be in. Once again, you're really two coaches. In the early stages, you'll be a disciplinarian, calling for precision and intentional focus. "Okay, do it again, but slower this time…. Good, now do it again." This foundation is vital, but there will also come a day when the neuroplasticity begins to take effect, and you'll look to become another kind of teacher entirely; a gentler and more permissive advocate for *wu wei:* "Just try softer" you might say. Or, maybe even better, "Don't try at all. Trust your body and let the movements come forth."

POSTURE, STANCE AND EQUIPOISE

No matter the style, martial art training also puts extraordinary emphasis on the physical fundamentals of posture and stance. Before we learn the first block, punch, or throw, we're instructed in the elemental practices of standing and walking in balance and equipoise. Think of your body as rooted in the ground, strong and stable through your legs and hips, yet flexible and adaptable in your arms and shoulders. You can't predict where an attack might come from or how it might develop, so it's best to be both strong and light, both stable and soft. Your posture should be proud but not arrogant; alert and awake but calm. Think of a bamboo plant that's both strong and flexible, able to withstand high winds.

This is equipoise. Balance in posture, balance in movement, and balance in spirit, always with the potential and the willingness to adapt on the fly. It's the perfect stance for combat but also for any encounter with an ambiguous and challenging world. You never know how an adversary might attack or move, so it's best to be both powerful and fluid. It's an ideal lesson for our encounters with a dynamic and increasingly incoherent modern world. In the near-term future, assaults on our sense of normality may come without warning and, in this sense, all of us will be called to martial artistry. If we're to survive, equipoise and equanimity will be essential.

THINKING WITH THE WHOLE BODY

Universally, martial art culture also embraces the idea of *embodied cognition*, the notion that intelligence is distributed across the entire body. In the modern West, a popular view holds that the mind is located inside the skull and that the rest of the body is little more than a locomotor device for the head. But in fact, it's all one thing: the body is always talking to the brain via movement, sensation, myokines, and other informational substances. It's not an exaggeration to say that we think with the whole body. When we move the body in intentional ways, we don't just train muscle, we train entire neural circuits. In this, martial art training—all Eastern disciplines in fact—stands in radical contrast to the "brain on a stick" approach that's so common in Western education.

In fact, the body is one thing and the brain—impressive as it is—will always be a subset of the body. Inevitably, the experience of the body will always influence the mind, cognition, and behavior. As Bessel van der Kolk has shown, this bottom-up approach is extremely powerful in transforming our mental states. We change, not by thinking, but by doing. In other words, experience is the driver; we transform through action. As some quipster has put it, "It's easier to act your way into a new way of thinking than it is to think your way into a new way of acting."

No one knows the power of this embodied, bottom-up approach better than thousands of "Karate Moms" across the modern world. We've heard the story again and again: The young child is bouncing off the walls, unruly, impulsive, and uncontrollable. At the end of her wits, Mom brings the offending creature to the local karate school and begs the sensei to bring some order to her life.

Sensei accepts the challenge, and over the course of the next several months, the process unfolds with simplicity, regularity, and disciplined physicality. "Bow to the mat. Kneel down before class begins. Sit quietly. Bow to the sensei. Bow to your training partner. Now, right leg back... Ready, punch!" The student repeats the pattern thousands of times and before long, Mom begins to notice a difference. The child is no longer so unruly; she seems calmer, more focused, more regulated, and more integrated. None of this is coincidence; work the body with disciplined precision and behavior is sure to follow.

We see a similar process in other physical domains. School teachers have long understood that handwriting solidifies student understanding of their lessons. The very act of holding a pencil and forming the letters has a profound effect on the brain and cognition. In fact, a solid body of research shows that when students take notes by hand, they walk away with a deeper understanding of the material than students who type on keyboards. The lesson here is simple: if you really want to drive your understanding home, bring your entire body into full participation.

FOCUS AND ATTENTION

Embodied cognition is fundamental to martial art training, but so too is the emphasis on concentration. "Pay attention, Grasshopper! Pay attention to your stance, your posture, your surroundings, and most of all, your training partner!" Not matter the particular fighting style, the focus is always on focus.

A thousand years before the discoveries of neuroscience, the ancients understood the importance of concentration in skill development and performance. Every teacher and school has its own methods and techniques, but the details don't matter much. The objective is full attention, sometimes described as *zanshin*, the state of spirit, mental alertness, and physical readiness to meet a combat or a defensive situation.

In feudal Japan, this state was intentionally cultivated not only in the dojo or training hall, but was held as a virtue across society, in all disciplines. In modern martial art programs, *zanshin* is still taught with the reminder "always train as if you're facing a live blade." An opponent with a razor-sharp sword is sure to get your attention.

In some respects, *zanshin* is similar to flow, that state of total immersion famously described by psychologist Mihály Csíkszentmihályi in the 1970s. In essence, flow is characterized by complete absorption in a task, energized focus, and full involvement. Csíkszentmihályi called this the Zone of Optimal Functioning.

残心

But no matter what we call it, we make a similar mistake in our approach. Here in the modern West, we're inclined to think of these mental states as some kind of special aptitude; you're either capable of intense focus and concentration in your sport or art, or you aren't.

But just as we saw in our conversation about neuroplasticity, we miss the fact that *zanshin* is an aptitude like any other and is thus trainable. In other words, *zanshin* is a muscle. Flow is a muscle. These mental states are a product of neurological circuitry, and these circuits can either wire together or fall apart, depending on how they're used.

In other words, we get better at radical awareness by practicing radical awareness. There might be some genetic or cultural influence that makes the process slightly easier, but this is very much beside the point. The way to develop *zanshin* is by practicing *zanshin*. In other words, put your students, athletes, and clients on task, and keep them there as long as possible.

MINIMALISM

Building a sense of equipoise is an essential part of experiential design, but the martial art model also provides an extremely useful aesthetic and guide for simple, minimalistic living. This begins in the traditional dojo, where cleanliness and order are held as high values; the training mat should be clean and swept daily, training tools and weapons must be kept in their proper places, and training uniforms must be clean and neat.

It's an elegant look, but this is about much more than superficial appearance or style. The ancient masters knew a great deal about human attention and they wanted their students to engage with deep focus. When people are swinging swords or practicing hand-to-hand combat, there's no room for distraction. A training environment that's simple, clean, and orderly makes it easier to concentrate on the present moment.

All of which can serve us well in the modern world. Fed up with the deluge of consumerism and the rising tide of junk that comes into our lives, more and more people are opting to go the other direction entirely. Sometimes billed as "voluntary simplicity," this approach serves as an antidote to stress, cognitive overload, and the general complexification of the modern world. In short, minimalism looks to create an island of sanity in a world that seems to be going off the rails.

Minimalism also aligns with a powerful ethic developed in the world of rock and alpine climbing. Beginning in the 1960s, climbers began to realize that conventional, expedition-style climbing was too laborious, too slow, and not really as adventurous as one might hope. In particular, Yvon Chouinard, the founder of Patagonia, emerged as an outspoken leader and advocate for better tools, lighter gear, and a more audacious approach to climbing the steep faces of Yosemite and the big mountains around the world.

Like the great Zen masters, Chouinard understood the importance of simplicity and means over ends. These days, any fool with enough equipment can get to the summit, but as he put it, "How you climb a mountain is more important than reaching the top." This insight led to a burst of innovation and a complete reassessment of the modern climber's relationship with stuff. Suddenly, the challenge was to own less gear and use it in more creative ways, a practice that's perfectly consistent with traditional martial art training. Don't clutter your dojo, your sport, or your life with superfluous possessions; concentrate on the fundamentals of what you're trying to do.

Of course, the prospect of minimalism or alpine style strikes many modern consumers as unappealing and unacceptable. Conditioned by decades of relentless marketing and advertising, we've come to expect and demand more and more of everything in our lives; making do with less feels diminishing. But minimalism isn't about scarcity or deprivation at all. Quite the opposite, it's really about abundance. Having less gives us the opportunity to be more, to do more, to feel more, to learn more.

In other words, don't focus on deprivation; focus on what minimalism makes possible. Look for solutions and possessions that are, in free-climber Alex Honnold's words, "radically adequate." Look for the affluence that comes with owning less.

Likewise, make your experiential design as simple and elegant as possible. It's tempting to deliver every possible experience and nuanced teaching to your students, clients, and athletes, but they're already drowning in complexity as it is. Instead, give them something clean, simple, orderly, and radically focused. Remember the words of Zen philosopher Alan Watts:

> The truth is revealed by removing things which stand in its light, an art, not unlike sculpture, in which the artist creates, not by building, but by hacking away.

TOUCH AND RESONANCE

There's yet another powerful benefit that comes from the martial art model: our direct, physical, and social contact with one another in practice, learning how other bodies move and respond to touch. It's particularly relevant at this moment in history because, tragically, the experience of interpersonal touch seems to be dying out. As the digital world comes to dominate our lives, we spend less and less time in authentic, face-to-face encounters and consequently, many of us are touch-deprived. Modern children often grow up with little experience in working with or playing with other human bodies, and tragically, our ability to sense and feel one another through touch is beginning to atrophy.

Clearly, today's students and young people need some remedial education in this practice, and martial art—like dance, theater, and other body-based disciplines—can provide this experience. Even simple games and drills can focus our attention on one another's posture, momentum, and facial expressions. Free from distraction, we can have a direct, felt experience of another person's disposition, their stance, and even their intention. We learn to speak, as some have put it, in "the language before words."

All of which aligns perfectly with discoveries in social neuroscience. In *The Neurobiology of We*, psychiatrist Daniel Siegel describes a "resonance circuit" that mediates the preverbal continuity and communication between human bodies. In a drastically simplified form, it goes like this: As we observe the movements, postures, eye movements, and microexpressions of other people's bodies and faces, we become sensitive to the pace of their conversation and their tone of voice, intonation, stress, and rhythm—the so-called prosody of communication. This information is processed by mirror neurons in the cortex of the brain, relayed downward through the limbic, emotional brain centers, and deep into the observer's body, where it's experienced as a gut feeling.

In effect, this circuitry allows us to run internal simulations of what other people are experiencing. When the system works properly, we get to feel what others are feeling and conversations tend to unfold smoothly. We understand one another and we feel felt. But when this resonance circuit atrophies through disuse or neglect, trouble is sure to follow. Communication disintegrates and people begin to feel isolated, lonely, and confused. We get frustrated with one another and conflict simmers. We attempt to compensate and connect via our devices, but there can be no substitute for actual physical encounters. If anything, our devices only make our suffering worse.

The solution lies in getting people back into physical contact with one another. We can do this through traditional combative drills, but we are also free to invent games and simple practices that demand attention and encourage safe touch. A background in the traditional martial arts will be helpful, but there's nothing to say that you can't innovate new practices of your own.

DOJO RULES

There's yet another powerful teaching that comes from the martial art model, one that sets us up for creating programs and cultures of excellence. Around the world, almost every martial art training program is built on some version of "dojo rules," time-honored guidelines for behavior in the training studio.

The rules vary in their details but are always centered around the importance of respect for people, process, and place. In short, students are expected to behave with honor, sincerity, and dignity in relationship to the people involved, the learning process, and the dojo itself. The typical set includes:

- Keep the training hall clean and orderly.

- Participate completely. Do not arrive late or leave early.

- Everyone trains with everyone else.

- Come to training with an empty cup, ready to learn.

These rules work because they create explicit behavioral guardrails and expectations. They make it clear: This experience is special. This is not a nightclub. This is not a movie theater. This is not a shopping center. This is a place to focus, concentrate, and deliver your best possible performance every day. This is a special place, home to a special experience that's worth protecting.

In turn, the rules set participants up for an experience that's focused, intentional, and roughly predictable. The body understands: Bow to the mat, bow to your partner, pay attention. The experience does the teaching. Students can relax into focused concentration and playful engagement. Even better, clear rules make it possible for us to play and train at a higher level.

The dojo rules are universal in the world of traditional martial art, but we see a similar emphasis in other domains, including the world of sport. In particular, we see it in the work of legendary basketball coach John Wooden. In fact, Wooden's programs showed an uncanny resemblance to martial art training in tone and emphasis. Wooden was a stickler on simple things like being on time for practice and presenting a neat and clean appearance.

Upon arriving at UCLA in the late 1940's, Wooden sent a multi-page memo to his players and staff, outlining his expectations for practice. The "Wooden's Rules" list is exhaustive, but key points are perfectly aligned with the dojo rules. Among them:

- Be dressed, on the floor, and ready for practice on time every day.

- Work hard to improve yourself without having to be forced. Be serious. Have fun without clowning. You develop only by doing your best.

- No cliques, no complaining, no criticizing, no jealousy, no egotism, no envy, no alibis. Earn the respect of all.

- When a coach blows the whistle, give your undivided attention and respond immediately.

- Take excellent care of your equipment and keep your locker neat and orderly.

- Do things the way you have been told. Correct habits are formed only through continuous repetition of the perfect model.

In describing Wooden's philosophy and success, NBA All-Star Bill Walton put it simply: "A culture of yes is built on a foundation of no." In other words, we get the best out of people by enforcing clear boundaries. By investing energy into focused practice sessions, Coach Wooden created habits of excellence that remained true, even under the stress of high-intensity playoff games. His players performed well in competition because they were accustomed to putting in their best effort every day.

No matter the domain, whether sport, martial art, education, or the workplace, explicit behavioral guidelines are essential in creating high-performance training environments. But sadly, our efforts are massively undercut by our consumer-centric culture of ease and convenience. Marketing professionals advise workshop leaders and trainers to make participation "as easy as possible." Pamper the customer, we're told; make it easy to sign up, easy to participate, easy to drop in, and easy to drop out. Relax your standards and cater to the whims of everyone.

But the end result is that the experience becomes diluted, devalued, and in some settings, nearly meaningless. Coach Wooden and every traditional sensei would be appalled by this wholesale watering down of our practices. And in this sense, our experiential designs need to be intentionally and explicitly counter-cultural. Teachers, coaches, and trainers must hold the line against the scourge of convenience; in the end, it's better to have a small number of dedicated participants than a shallow program of partial engagement.

Of course, none of this is easy. As teachers, trainers, coaches, and parents, some of us are slow to enforce rules of any kind, especially when we're just getting started in a leadership role. Many of us are conflict averse and we don't like telling other people what to do. We want to be friendly and easygoing, and if someone behaves badly, our inclination is to let it go and hope that the perpetrator corrects her behavior, or that others will step in with some kind of enforcement.

But this laissez-faire attitude is actually a recipe for greater friction and conflict in the long run, not to mention a degradation of the experience itself. Consistent, even-handed enforcement sends a message that "this experience is valuable and worth protecting." So be a stickler. Eventually, people will understand that this experience is an island of sanity in a world of noise and distraction. By enforcing the rules consistently and fairly, you'll build a space of quality, focus, humanity, and excellence. Enforce the rules and you'll create something special, maybe even something sacred.

THE WEST AFRICAN DRUM AND DANCE MODEL

> It would be reasonable to say that everything that happens in our bodies is rhythmic until proven otherwise.
>
> —Josephine Arendt, neurobiologist

> "Adabakadi! Adabakadi! Good morning, good afternoon, good evening! Welcome to our circle."

So goes a traditional greeting of West African drum and dance culture, our next inspirational model for experiential design and high-functioning humans. A true cultural masterpiece, the drum circle is an ideal practice for helping people grow and thrive. There's rhythm, physicality, community, and a real sense of inclusion. It's a proven method and there's no surprise that drumming has become increasingly popular around the modern world. In schools, and even in the workplace, drum circles are now widely embraced not just as fun and engaging musical events but as a powerful whole-body method for promoting health and building community.

The beauty of drumming and in fact, any rhythmic activity, is that it serves as an experiential antidote to our modern state of distress and arrythmia. As many of us are coming to recognize, modern life has become increasingly chronic, static, and stagnant; a flat-line, high-stress experience in a world that's intrinsically dynamic.

Beginning with the obliteration of circadian rhythm by artificial light, modern humans have been leveling out almost every rhythmic process in the natural world. Seasonal rhythms, nutritional rhythms, work and rest rhythms, and even our conversational rhythms have been crushed by always-on technology and 24/7 commerce. In short, nobody feels much of a swing anymore; it's all one grinding, never-ending slog that degrades and diminishes the vitality of the human animal.

But when we drum, we experience an intimate physical reminder of the deep oscillations that animate the lives of every living being. Not only do we feel it in our bodies, we also get the metaphor and the message that goes with it. That is, there's a waxing and a waning to everything, a rising and a falling of energy and experience. We relax into the process, knowing that even if we're awkward and out of step with the rest of the music, all we have to do is wait a bit. The rhythm will come around again and we can rejoin the action when the time is right. In the process, we feel a sense of relief. No longer do we need to strive in every moment; once we feel the beat, our bodies know what they need to do.

Likewise, the physical benefits are easy to understand and appreciate. Just as with sport or any other highly focused activity, drumming concentrates the body in a single cohesive effort; it integrates the kludge of various subsystems into a single whole. It releases endorphins, enkephalins, endogenous opiates, and alpha waves in the brain, all of which are associated with feelings of well-being and euphoria. Not surprisingly, studies show a decrease in stress and pain. Drumming might even boost immunity and the production of natural T-cells, which help the body combat cancer as well as other diseases.

Clearly, this is about a lot more than hands in motion. To lay down a coherent beat, we've got to invite the entire body to the process. And in this dialogue, the body tends to unify all of its energies. The movement of the hands brings order to our bodies, our physiology, and our spirits, but the voice works a kind of magic as well. To a degree not seen in other musical arts, West African drum culture puts enormous emphasis on singing the beats we're trying to play. It's not enough to simply listen and repeat; to really own the rhythm and the pattern, you've got to vocalize it.

A classic example is a popular djembe accompaniment *moribayassa*. Your teacher will ask students to vocalize it by saying out loud, "ba da bity ba, ba da bity ba..." Repeat it back, over and over until it sinks into your body, then let your their hands take over. Or, you can simply say the names of the notes out loud, "slap-slap, tone-tone-slap," and so on. For beginners, it feels awkward and many of us are shy about singing of any kind, but the process is almost magical in its effectiveness. Singing comes from the deep body and, in turn, helps guide the hands.

Drumming is about music obviously, but West African drum culture goes further in the way it encourages participation of entire communities. In some settings, a drum ensemble will play a show before a live audience, but even in a performance, spectators are encouraged to join in with singing and dancing; historically speaking, it's an event for the entire village.

All of which stands in sharp contrast to our modern entertainment-centric culture. Beginning with the age of television, vital elements of the human experience—music, singing, dance, and sports—were transformed from something that people did to something that people watched. In other words, an entire range of human activity that used to be participatory is now observed at arm's length. Specialists and experts showcase their arts with impressive skill, leaving us fascinated by their performances, but the experience of passive observation just doesn't take us very far. In the end, it's participation that really moves and transforms us. Participation, we might say, is the secret of life.

ABORIGINAL VALUES AND HISTORY

When it comes to the history of drum culture, we don't really know how the whole thing began. Some say that the *djembe* drum was invented in the twelfth century, but documentation is scarce and it's safe to assume that our ancestors were more interested in practicing their music than in leaving a written trail for us to follow.

Geographically, the traditional distribution of the *djembe* is associated with the Mali Empire, and included parts of the modern-day countries of Guinea, Mali, Burkina Faso, Ivory Coast, Gambia, and Senegal. According to the Bambara people in Mali, the name "djembe" comes from the saying "Anke djé, anke bé," meaning "everyone gather together in peace."

But whatever the historical details, we can be certain that West African drum and dance culture emerged from the indigenous, aboriginal, native worldview. In this culture, all things connect and all is relationship. For native Africans and most indigenous people as well, matter and spirit are considered to be complementary and in constant dialogue with one another. Matter speaks to spirit, spirit speaks to matter. There is no separation.

Likewise, we also see a strong emphasis on reciprocity, conversation, and dialogue. The acts of giving and receiving are fundamental to all life and are implicit in the act of drumming. The teacher issues a "call" and the student attempts to answer with a "response."

This musical give-and-take is particularly notable in advanced drum ensembles, where individual players "speak" to one another in a way that resembles our familiar spoken language. Solo voices and instruments are all well and good, but expression is even more interesting in conversation with others. In fact, West Africans would surely agree with the poet Rumi: "Human beings are discourse. Everything is conversation." This is a vital lesson that modern people might well take to heart; as rich and meaningful conversation becomes increasingly endangered, we need all the reminders we can get.

But drumming, especially in the West African tradition, goes even further, deep into the psycho-spiritual realm. It's music to be sure, but it's also a way to access unseen regions of the life experience, the world of energy and imagination. In modern conversations about drumming and dance, there's a great deal of talk about the neuroscience behind the experience, but for indigenous people, the experience was never about synapses, neurotransmitters, or particular regions of the brain; neurons have nothing to do with it. Instead, there's a powerful sense of extension and opening that comes when we merge with the beat. Feel the energy of the circle, relax into it, and allow yourself to become vulnerable to the vastness of the experience.

COMMUNITY

The individual benefits that come with drumming are all well and good, but the experience really stands out in the way that it builds a genuine sense of community. Many drum gatherings begin with the greeting *wantanara*: "We are one." It's a great aspiration and, in an age of rampant individualism and narcissism, stands as a promising antidote for our alienation and loneliness.

Like the team sport experience we saw earlier, group drumming has a powerful bonding effect, driven by the shared predicament of music making. Everyone in the circle is struggling together to get it right, everyone is making mistakes, everyone is teetering on the edge of grasping the rhythms or losing the beat entirely. There's a palpable sense of unity in this effort; as nervous systems fire together, minds and bodies wire together.

In fact, we can think of a drum ensemble as a kind of

dynamic tensegrity structure, reminiscent of Buckminster Fuller's geodesic domes. In an ideal circumstance, everyone in the group would play with perfect execution, but mistakes are inevitable, even for advanced players. But error is rarely catastrophic because every player leans on others for rhythmic cues. If someone's play is weak, other players will pick up the slack. The rhythm is a shared creation.

Likewise, we're reminded of the African social orientation called *ubuntu*. Strictly speaking, the word *ubuntu* comes from the indigenous tradition of South Africa, but a similar orientation runs throughout drum and dance culture. In this worldview, personal identity is always tied to the welfare of the group, tribe, and community. As the saying goes: "I am who I am because of who we are." And in the words of Desmond Tutu, "You can't be human on your own."

In the modern West, *ubuntu* is sometimes described as team spirit, and it's not unusual for athletic coaches to use this language in promoting team unity. But in the indigenous tradition, *ubuntu* runs far deeper than any sporting vibe. In the modern Western world, athletic teams are transient and constantly in flux. Especially at the pro level, team alliances are always shifting as players are traded, get injured, or retire. In other words, team spirit is tenuous, provisional, and symbolic; loyalties shift like the wind. But in its original form, *ubuntu* is rooted in actual lived experience, as tribes and villages are bound together by the literal need to survive; if the tribe fails, everyone fails. This is a dead-serious orientation.

All of which sounds good on its face, but drumming is a lot more than just a warm and fuzzy feel-good, prosocial experience. The *ubuntu* orientation also serves as a powerful antidote to the steep pyramid of inequality and hierarchy that defines the modern world. In other words, it's practically vital in our efforts to create a functional future. To put it yet another way, equality doesn't just feel better, it actually works better.

This is precisely the point of *The Spirit Level: Why Greater Equality Makes Societies Stronger*, by Richard Wilkinson and Kate Pickett. The authors argue that inequality erodes trust, while it increases anxiety, illness, and excessive consumption. Across a broad range of social conditions, outcomes are significantly worse in more unequal societies: physical and mental health, drug abuse, education, imprisonment, obesity, social mobility, community life, violence, teen pregnancy, and child well-being. To put it another way, inequality is a powerful driver of social dysfunction and it's bad for everyone. Even if we somehow manage to claw our way to a position of power and wealth, we're still living in a dysfunctional community.

This is where drumming comes in. By aligning our experience and our neurobiology together in a shared effort, we leave hierarchy behind, at least for a moment. The drum circle may not spread the wealth or power in the world at large but, at the very least, it gives us a precious sense of unity and reminds us of our universal humanity: "We are people through other people."

SKILL DEVELOPMENT

Even beyond its powerful community-building benefits, drumming also offers us a handy model, even a laboratory of sorts, for exploring the fundamentals of skill development and training. One drum, two hands, three notes (bass, tone, slap); the simplicity serves us well. If we can learn on such an elemental level, perhaps we can extend our understanding to more complex challenges and to learning in general.

Just as we've seen in the worlds of athletic training and martial art, West African drum training offers a perfect example of quality reps. Deep, immersive practice and focused concentration are the key ingredients here, and there are few distractions in the circle. The teacher lays down a pattern and everyone attempts to repeat it. Call and response, over and over again. Listen with your "big ear" and feel the beat resonate in your body. Play the rhythms as best you can, repeat until the point of awkwardness, then go home and sleep as deeply as possible. When you wake up the next day, you'll be pleasantly surprised to feel a new sense of ease and competence. This is neuroplasticity in action.

In one sense, it's easy; just put in the reps and the skill will come. But drum training is about more than simple patterns with the hands. In essence, it's really about attentional training and focus. We lay down a familiar beat and play for a while, but then the mind begins to wander and we fall out of sync. We make a clumsy mistake, then pull our attention and our hands back into rhythm. In this sense, drum training has a great deal in common with familiar forms of meditation. Choose a target—typically the breath—stay on task as best you can, but when the mind wanders, bring it back. Drumming is no different.

In fact, the process of learning to drum is perfectly consistent with what we know about the neurobiology of attention and skill development. In particular, it's a vivid example of the top-down flow of neural processing. When we learn a new rhythm, we start with conscious intention, working at the level of the brain's cortex. "I'm going to play a tone with my right hand, then a bass note with my left," and so on. It's all very scripted and disciplined. We do our best to get it right, just like our teacher asked.

Next, we do the reps: thousands of quality, intentional, highly focused reps, with practice sessions broken up by rest and sleep. Keep this rhythm going for a few weeks or months and almost magically, the neurological activity in your cortex begins to settle into the deeper, more primal regions of your brain: especially the limbic system and the hippocampus. From there, the patterns are absorbed by your hands and arms in the form of muscle memory. Now you've got your body into the act and, with additional practice, you can relax into a genuine musical expression.

At this point, your teacher is likely to tell you "Don't think...feel." Let go of your conscious striving and let your body take over. "Try softer." Relinquish the effort. Trust your body to get it right. Allow the rhythm to come forth. You've heard the beat a thousand times and your internal metronome knows what to do. The "I" fades away as you relax into effortless action and the realm of *wu wei*.

To put it another way, drum practice offers a particularly vivid example of rhythmic oscillation between freedom and discipline in training. In the discipline phase, the teacher puts a strong emphasis on playing patterns in a very particular way. There's a right way to play *fanga*, *kakilambe*, or *yankadi*, for example. Regional differences exist, but nevertheless, there's a right way and a wrong way to play these accompaniments. For the student, this phase is all about focus and discipline. It's demanding, even exhausting. Stay focused and keep doing the reps until you get it just so.

This discipline is vital, but there's also a complementary phase that's all about letting go into emotion and improv. Just play; let your body do what it wants to do. And in this phase, as jazz musician Miles Davis famously put it, "There are no wrong notes." Errors are simply stepping stones to the unfolding pattern, so keep moving; get out of the way and let your body do what it wants to do. This is where the magic happens. When we let go, it feels like the instrument (the body) plays itself. As effort dissipates, the musician merges with the music. Even better, the musician disappears almost entirely, and the music takes on a life of its own.

PLAY A BEAT YOU CAN REPEAT

There's yet another benefit that comes to us on our drumming journey and that's the way it nudges us into a state of humility and good humor. Learning a basic rhythm looks like the easiest thing in the world, but we mess up more often than we'd like. We're astounded that we can't get our hands to do what we want and even the smallest drift in attention leads to disaster. Even when we do get into the groove, our teacher is sure to add more layers of complexity. She wants us to tap our foot, pay attention to our breathing, and maybe even sing the beat out loud. And even worse, she wants us to reverse our handing to an ambidextrous, mirror-image pattern.

Every element is simple on its own, but when we try to put it all together, it quickly falls apart. It's frustrating and even maddening. How can something so simple be so incredibly difficult? But everyone in the circle is going through the same struggle and our teacher remembers full well what she had to go through on her journey. And there's nothing to be done about any of it, except to try again and laugh at our awkwardness and our shared predicament. There's a reason so many drummers are smiling and laughing when they play; they know full well how improbable the whole thing is.

YOU'VE GOT WHAT IT TAKES

In a perfect world, drum and dance would be an integral part of our experiential design. Likewise, it should be part of every school curriculum, beginning in elementary and extending deep into high school and beyond. But there are bound to be challenges. It's a big effort to round up drums for everyone in your group, and you'll have to be courteous to your neighbors; not everyone likes hearing the beat, even when it's skillful and musical.

But the biggest obstacle and most perplexing objection is the common belief that "I don't have rhythm." This is a popular claim among the inexperienced and it's really rather astonishing. To be sure, not everyone has worked with rhythm, and some of us pick it up faster than others, but the human animal is fully capable of finding and feeling a beat. Without question, this is a human universal. Almost every culture has some form of rhythmic engagement and, from a big human-history perspective, it's utterly normal and not even all that remarkable.

Everyone can imitate and feel a pulse. Just as we imitate one another's postures and facial expressions via mirror neurons in the brain's cortex, so too can we copy the beats laid down by a more advanced percussionist. This is the basis for spoken language and, in turn, musical training. Almost as soon as we're born, we start to repeat what we hear, copying and imitating words, tones, accents, and pace. It's a natural progression: hear it, copy it, play with it. We all do it; the only challenge is that we forget. As adults, we spend less time in imitation and, before long, some of us come to the astonishing conclusion that we just can't do it.

To be sure, learning to drum can feel like learning a foreign language; easy when we're young and more difficult as we get older. Nevertheless, the capacity never really goes away. What does go away is the willingness to fight our way through the incompetence, the awkwardness, and the embarrassment that comes with being a beginner again. But as we've seen, neuroplasticity is always at work in the background, rearranging circuits and tissue to create new aptitudes, skills, and competencies. And in this sense, the whole enterprise is actually quite straightforward. All you need to do is to keep showing up, keep trying, and trust the process. If you can tap your foot, you're on your way.

CHAPTER 7
EXECUTION

Use only that which works, and take it from any place you can find it.

—Bruce Lee

As you can see, our experiential design models give us plenty of inspiration, and you're probably excited to dig in and create something special, even magical for your people. Going back to our veterinarian model and the beginner's mind, you're thinking about objectives and how you might shape an experience to train high-functioning humans. You want something that's relevant and meaningful, friendly but challenging, disciplined but playful. You want to help your students, clients, and athletes interact with one another and maybe learn some new skills. Along the way, you'll want them to experience the sweet spot of stress and to trust in the magic of neuroplasticity. And maybe, if you work with them consistently, they'll get a taste of *wu wei*—that delicious state of skill, mastery, and effortless action. So given what you'd like to accomplish, what are the vital elements you'd like to include in the experience?

Naturally, your wish list will depend on your situation

and your resources. Ideally, you'd like to go all in on a deep immersion and get your people together for a long stretch in an idyllic retreat setting where everything is on tap for a profoundly pro-human, nature-based experience. But obviously, this is a big ask and it's rarely possible to do as much as we'd like. Ideally, we'd want to see that everyone gets lots of physical movement, social time, great food, great sleep, and sustained contact with the natural world, but this can be a heavy lift, and you'll surely have to make some compromises along the way.

Or, maybe your goals are more modest. Maybe you'd be happy to simply lead some basic classes for students, clients, patients, or athletes. You don't have the luxury of time or resources, but you're determined to create the best possible experience in the time you have. In any case, now would be a good time to take an in-depth look at some of the essential elements of experiential design.

THE ONE-HOUR MODEL

When it comes to planning the structure of your program and experiences, there are thousands of possible combinations of time, location, and activity. You've got a rough idea of how to put it all together, but you'll probably be constrained by conditions, resources, and the reality of people's lives.

The possibilities are sure to feel overwhelming at times, but for simplicity's sake, let's imagine a one-hour experience or, allowing for transitions, 50 minutes. This will give you a template to build on. Even if you're not planning on doing one-hour sessions with people, it's still a good reference point. If you can master a one-hour class, you can scale up as desired.

Once you feel confident with a one-hour session, you can use it as an expandable guide for longer experiences. Simply multiply the pattern to fit into a half day, full day, or multiple days. For example, two or three cycles makes for a solid half day event, four or five cycles for a full day workshop, and so on.

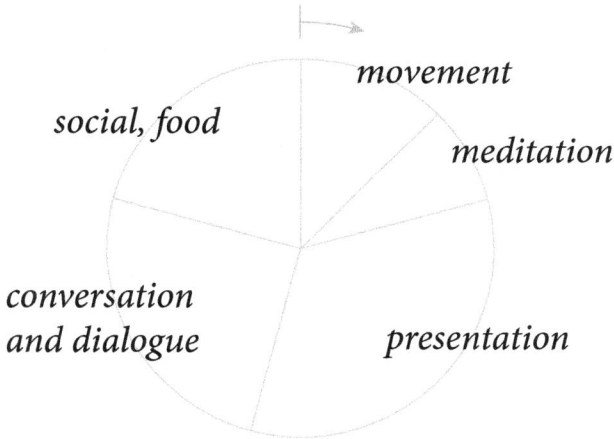

The beauty of this approach is that it provides a predictable rhythm both for you and your people. Working with the one hour model, everyone knows what's coming. One-hour sessions also work well because they seem to fit the typical attention span of most people. There's some highly focused engagement, then some time for rest, social time, bathroom breaks, and so on. There's a beat to it; a beat you can repeat.

Naturally, you'll design your one-hour model to suit your purposes, but for now, let's assume common elements of movement, meditation, presentation, and social time. Depending on your objectives, you might include more or less movement, more or less presentation, more or less meditation, and so on. The details don't matter as long as you stick to the fundamental rhythm.

Adjust the proportions as desired but be sure to consider the sequence. That is, no matter the setting, it makes good sense to start with the body, with movement and meditation. It's always safe to assume that your people are in need of a physical refresher, so this is always a good place to begin. Simply adjust the time and proportions for each segment, taking deep dives or short snacks as desired.

Next up is your cognitive content and presentation. By now, your people should be feeling energized and attentive, so your words and ideas should be well received. Take whatever time you need with this segment but avoid the "long wind." Stick to the essential points and keep it focused. As your presentation concludes, you'll have some options. Ideally, people will have questions and curiosities; this will be a good time for conversation, so build this into your experience. And of course, this leads naturally into a break, casual social time, and food.

As you'll see, this template works wonders for keeping people focused, alert, and engaged. In other words, the experience feeds the whole human animal. There's physical engagement, stillness in meditation, cognitive stimulation, and plenty of opportunity for conversation and discussion. No matter your particular domain or discipline, this is a model that works.

MOVEMENT

Without question, the most primal element will always

be physical movement. As most everyone knows, movement—aka "exercise"—primes the body and the mind for engagement and makes everything else go better. Moving our bodies gives us a deep sense of control, which in turn helps us relax and feel at home in the world. The practice promotes brain health and gives us an opportunity to express ourselves and our emotions. And even better, it's just plain fun. This is a time for discovery, celebration, and expression; it's a time to honor our animal nature.

There are lots of ways you can integrate this practice into your design. It might be a robust centerpiece of your program, or it can be a supplement that enhances everything else that you might be doing. Your movement sessions might be sustained, sweaty periods of deep engagement, or they might span just a few minutes; it all depends on your objectives, your time, and your setting.

Of course, you might encounter an obstacle right at the outset: Maybe you're not, strictly speaking, qualified to teach physical movement. In today's legalistic environment, a common assumption holds that anyone who aspires to teach "exercise" should have a professional qualification and certification. We assume that there's an essential body of knowledge involved, usually the science of anatomy, biomechanics, and physiology. Likewise, a deeper, often unspoken assumption holds that physical movement is inherently dangerous and injury-promoting, often expressed in the ominous warning, "Before beginning an exercise program, see your doctor."

But in fact, the human animal is deeply wired for vigorous movement. Physical activity is not just historically normal, it's almost universally health promoting. Almost every form of movement succeeds in improving the health of the human animal, and in most practices, injuries are rare. People have been teaching dance and sport for hundreds if not thousands of years, and in the overwhelming majority of cases, the result is almost always positive. In other words, there's no reason to be afraid of teaching movement. Yes, it's possible that some people will get injured in the process, but expert knowledge is no guarantee either; even with professional supervision, people still get hurt on occasion.

So even if you're not a trainer or a movement teacher, you can still step up with some basic leadership. Even a simple movement session—a few minutes of calisthenics or jogging in place—led by an average person, is better than nothing. In fact, we might even say that it's even *better* than expert instruction. Movement leadership by a nonspecialist normalizes the practice and sends a powerful message: This experience is too important to be left to experts. We all need to move, even in circumstances that might be less than ideal.

Likewise, some of us will be distracted by the myth of perfect form. We've been conditioned to believe that there are ideal movement patterns that we must adhere to and that failure to follow these perfect forms will inevitably lead to injury. But when we look at the vast individual differences between human bodies and, in particular, our widely divergent personal histories, both good and bad, it becomes more and more difficult to point to any biomechanical ideal that works for everyone.

In fact, when it comes to teaching human movement, it's close to being the case that, to paraphrase Miles Davis, "There are no wrong moves." The body is capable of millions of movement combinations, and in the vast majority of instances, all of it is health promoting. So there's no reason to be afraid. Just be sensible. Start slow, ease people into it, encourage a strong effort, and remind your people to back off if something doesn't feel right. To be sure, if your goal is a particular clinical outcome or expert performance in a particular sport, sophisticated knowledge is essential. But for most people, most of the time, almost any vigorous movement will give you the desired result: happier, more alert and engaged human animals.

MOVEMENT SNACKS

Big sweaty movement sessions are fantastic, but there's also enormous value in brief sessions of light movement, what some people call "movement snacks." The idea here is not to develop robust fitness or train people for competitive sporting events but rather to help people sustain their connection with the body and refresh their sense of physicality. These mini sessions provide an essential break from the grinding cognitive work that has come to dominate our modern lives.

All you need is a small open area, indoors or out. A few minutes of arm swings, squats, and lunges will bring your body-mind back into integration. You'll get your breathing turned on and your metabolism up and running. For best results, repeat often. A short movement snack every couple of hours or so is perfectly appropriate in almost any setting.

In any case, the point is to feel help your people feel their animal vitality. In the process, you'll re-establish the mind-body unity that's been disrupted by the acute or chronic stress experience of our modern, alien environment. In this sense, it doesn't matter how many calories people are burning or what their heart rate happens to be. It doesn't matter what kind of shoes they're wearing, how fast they're going, how much they're lifting, or what their electronic device has to say about it all. What matters is how people *feel*. If you can promote the signal of a strong, vigorous animal body in action, you're doing it right.

Likewise, it doesn't really matter what kind of equipment you happen to have on hand. Use whatever you've got and don't be distracted by the belief that you need expensive gadgets, machines, or devices. In fact, you can do a comprehensive, even demanding session with body weight, motion, and gravity. Remember, the human body has a long history of vigorous movement in wild, outdoor habitats, completely free from clipboards, iPads, heart rate monitors, or other gizmos. And nonhuman animals in the wild seem to do just fine with, well, nothing.

So, if you've got dumbbells, use 'em. If you've got physioballs, sticks, ropes, ladders, sandbags, or rocks, use 'em. If you've got stairs, run or walk 'em. That said, there's one exception to this minimalist approach: the medicine ball. The beauty of medicine balls is that they're fun and super versatile. There are hundreds of possible movement combinations and social games that you can try. And because they're free weights, medicine balls provide functional training with real-world objects. Even better, they're great for practical core conditioning and they last forever.

THEMES AND COACHING PROMPTS

When selecting moves for your students, clients, children, or patients, it's easy to be intimidated by the myriad possibilities. There's so much to choose from and to make matters worse, there are thousands of divergent opinions on what makes for an ideal movement or training session. Fortunately, you don't have to nail down everything or come up with perfect routines. In most cases, all you really need is a simple set of themes and coaching prompts.

As always, concentrate on function. Forget about appearance and put your focus on movement, not muscles. Some people will be intimidated and some will even be ashamed of their physical condition, so put them at ease by taking the spotlight off appearance. Don't talk about weight loss, toning, or sculpting. Instead, focus on the fundamentals of basic movement: how to stand, how to reach, how to get up off the floor, how to lift an object. Look for moves that are multi-joint and multi-plane. Look for moves that are consistent with locomotion and human evolution. Look for moves that are fun and graceful.

In particular, emphasize upright posture and extension through the torso and spine. This is a common theme in the dance world and is a powerful antidote to our modern experience of chronic flexion, with forward head posture and compressed, inhibited breathing through the diaphragm and abdomen.

In contrast, extension rebalances posture, invigorates the spine, and promotes deeper breathing. You can promote this with a variety of simple moves, especially high reaches. Stand tall, be proud, move smoothly and gracefully. We're all aspiring athletes and dancers here.

It's also a good idea to emphasize multi-plane movement variations. Living in a culture of workish productivity as

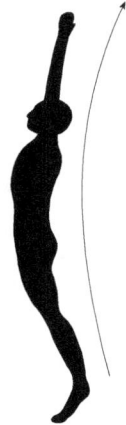

we do, we often fall into the habit of relentless forward movement and linear patterns in the sagittal plane. We're dedicated to action and we want to get things done, all of which is reflected in the way we move our bodies.

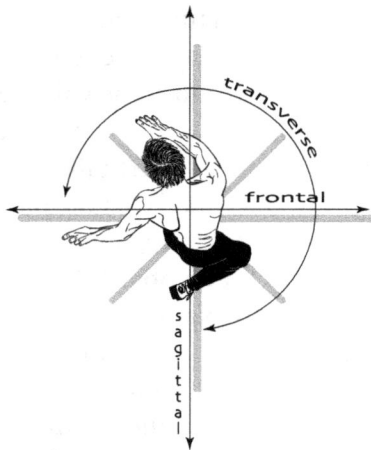

But the human animal thrives on rotational movement in the transverse plane. Muscles, tendons, joints, and spinal discs are nourished by diverse, dance-like moves. And in particular, the nervous system and brain enjoy the stimulation that comes when we cross the centerline of the body in cross-body reaches and rotation; switching between left and right brain hemispheres seems to have an almost magical effect.

No matter which particular movements you choose, a set of general principles will serve you well. As you lead your movement sessions, coach your people with prompts that emphasize whole-body integration and sensation:

"Solid stances, people!"

"Bend your knees!"

"Feel your feet on the ground, feel your legs, feel your breath."

"Get your whole body involved! Hips talk to shoulders! Toenails to fingernails!"

"Move from your center, your *hara*, your *tan tien*."

"Slow down and focus on the fundamentals. Remember, slow is smooth, smooth is fast."

"Motion is lotion."

"Feel what you're feeling."

"Keep adjusting. If something hurts, stop doing it or do something else."

SOLO MOVES

The simplest way to lead your movement session is to start with the familiar format: The teacher or coach stands in front of class, demonstrates a movement, and invites everyone to try it for themselves. And naturally, most of us will assume that the place to begin is with some kind of "warm-up." We've seen it and experienced it a million times, and it seems to make sense.

But what we're really after here is something a bit more nuanced, described with the word *thixotropy*. It's a fancy word, but the principle is easy to understand; some substances become more liquefied with agitation: think of clay, paint, liquid concrete, and even mountain slopes. Officially, these materials are described as "non-Newtonian" substances; they're solid, but once they're moved, stretched, or shaken they become more liquid.

What's fascinating here is that human bodies have similar characteristics. In fact, almost every tissue in the body is thixotropic or non-Newtonian. Think of the cytoplasm in every cell. Think of cell membranes, fascia, muscles, tendons, and even organs. If we agitate these tissues with contractions, vibrations, stretching, or massage, they become more liquid and, in turn, metabolites and nutritional substances begin to flow freely. And this, of course, is the optimal state for health. To put it another way, liquid animals are healthy animals.

The good news is that it doesn't take much, nor does it have to follow some particular method or protocol. Simply jogging in place gets the thixotropy rolling. Stir things up or dance as desired. A few contractions, especially the big muscles of your legs and hips, a few easy stretches, and maybe some shaking and vibration, and your people will be good to go.

Arm swings

With this in mind, a good place to start is with standing arm swings. This pattern is easy, rhythmic, and nothing more than an exaggeration of the arm swings that we'd normally do in walking or running. It also speaks to the whole body. Once your people get moving, they'll begin to feel the sensation, deep into their torso, hips, and legs.

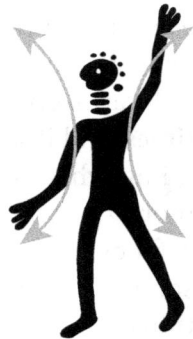

And don't let them be distracted by the fact that this is an "easy" move. Instead, work the variations as you call for diagonal arm swings or big arcs, including lateral rotation at the shoulders. You can also increase the demand by having your people do the whole series on one foot; it's functional, challenging, and athletic. Sustain this movement for a while and it won't be so easy anymore.

Backstroke, reaches, and flutter kicks

This is just what it sounds like: a dry-land version of what you might do in a swimming pool. Vary the speed, the angles, and in particular, the feeling of movement in the shoulder blades, (scapula) the back and rib cage.

Next, add some vertical reaches, looking for length through your the whole body. Vary the amplitude of the moves and the speed, encouraging people to reach higher, even on tiptoes. Don't quit early. Sustain the moves as long as comfortable, then have your people relax and notice the sensation. There's a good chance they'll feel noticeably taller.

Giant circles

Next up are giant circles, a serious challenge for balance and proprioception. Have your people stand on one foot and pretend they're drawing big circles, in any plane, including diagonals. You can call for circles in the sagittal plane, the frontal plane, and for the most advanced version, even a circle overhead. To increase the challenge, ask your people to slow down and smooth it out. This will get their attention!

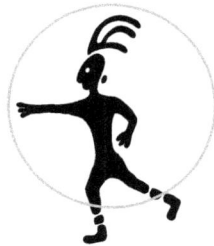

Solo shapes

As you'll discover, there are millions of possible move-ment combinations that you can explore, but you can keep things simple by using the shapes below. These are easy to remember and are appropriate for everyone, from begin-ners to elite athletes. Used in combination with various stances, steps, speeds, and sizes, these shapes will give you thousands of possible movement combinations. They also work great with a medicine ball.

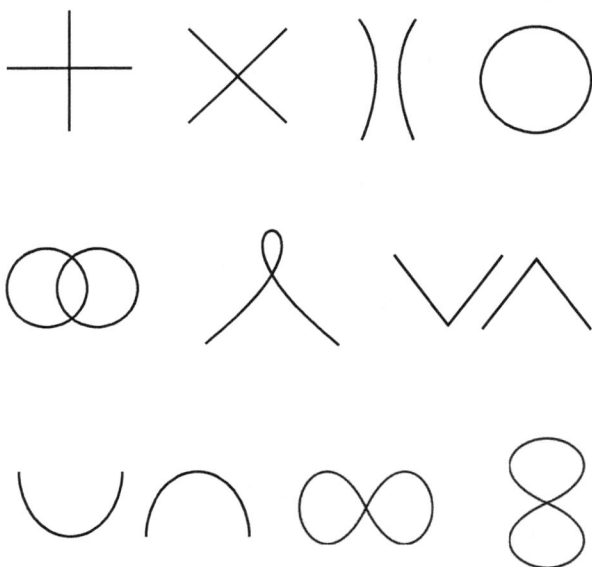

For example, pick a theme for the day. Let's say you're going to explore the simple diagonal lines. Start by tracing the basic shape, but don't stop there. Explore variations in amplitude, speed, and in particular, participation by the rest of the body, especially the hips and legs.

At first, these moves will feel ridiculously easy, but you can increase the challenge by adding some stance options. Work the same shapes and lines as before, but with one foot forward in a staggered stance. That's pretty easy, so go to one foot to amplify the challenge.

Next, work the diagonal lines while stepping forward, backward, or laterally. This will give you hundreds of possible moves that can be as easy or demanding as you like. If you're ambitious, you can even add hops and jumps.

The great thing about using these shapes is that there's not much to remember. Your students can simply refer back to the basic forms for their own movement snacks at home or in the workplace. Even better, many of these shapes appear in other physical disciplines such as dance and martial art. If you can master these moves, you'll be fluent in other arts as well.

SOCIAL RAPPORT

Solo movements are all well and good for individual conditioning, warm-ups, and somatic exploration, but the real action comes when we get people physically interacting with one another. Not only will your people get the benefit of vigorous movement, they'll also build trust and a sense of rapport. Try the following progression for best results:

Spotting

Begin with safety. As we've seen, the human animal needs to feel the friendliness of their world, and if we can ease their concerns about physical danger, people will begin to relax and play at a higher level. We build this sense of safety with spotting drills, commonly seen in gymnastic studios and even rock-climbing gyms. The idea here is to contain unstable movement, falls, and stumbles with your hands, arms, or body.

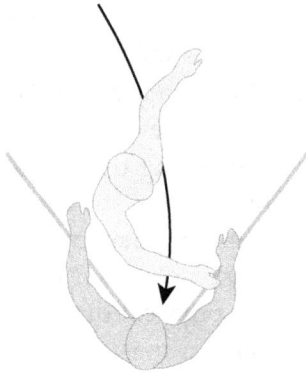

As a coach, show people how to protect one another with a strong stance and a funnel-like shape with your arms. When someone stumbles, protect them from falling by guiding them back into balance and safety. Use your hands and arms to manage their motion, keep them upright, and prevent them from crashing into obstacles. It's easy, but the very act of practice creates an atmosphere of safety and care. Practice this often, especially when new people come into your program.

Heckling and stance testing

Once people feel comfortable, the next step is heckling and stance testing. A *heckle* is simply a light, gentle nudge to your partner's shoulder, back, or hips; think of it as a balance and stability challenge. This is practical, functional athletic training that's also a lot of fun.

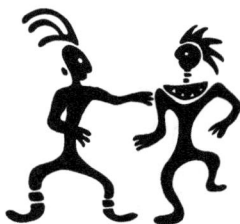

Instruct players to use a soft hand, shoulder, or hip to heckle their training partner, and have them try it in all three planes: sagittal, frontal, and transverse. Light heckles will stimulate proprioceptive sensitivity in your partner's feet, ankles, knees, and hips. Try this game in a variety of stances: normal standing, on one foot, and so on. When you've got rapport going, you can increase the intensity.

Next, work stance stability with light, targeted pushes to your partner's shoulder. First, concentrate on simple stability. Your partner receives the heckle and steps back into a strong stance, maintaining maximum integration through hips, torso, and upper body. Above all, don't fall down. Have people adjust their stances as necessary to absorb additional pushes.

Next, try fluidity. As the heckle or push contacts the shoulder, allow the shoulder to give way with no resistance. Stand firm or step as necessary, allowing your shoulder to yield like water.

Or have your players imagine that their torso is like a door on a hinge. When the push comes, allow the door to swing open easily and effortlessly. Repeat with a series of pushes and heckles.

Finally, mix the two responses as desired. It's your partner's choice: when the push comes, people can either be strong or fluid, but whatever the choice, make it a complete, athletic movement with full intention and whole-body integration. When you've got the rapport going, increase the intensity as desired.

As the action unfolds, you'll want to put a lot of emphasis on communication between training partners. Some people are shy about asking for what they need in these encounters, so be assertive and explicit in your instruction:

> "These games require physical negotiation and you'll be working with a broad range of people, so it's important to speak up. If your partner is moving too fast or slow for your taste, say so. If someone is being too strong, say so. If you want more intensity in the movement, say so."

In other words, don't assume anything. Be sure to demonstrate assertive behavior and communication; tell your partner "That's too much" or "Give me more." Make it clear that if people feel uncomfortable with any of these interactions or if something gives them pain, they're free to sit quietly at the perimeter of the training area. No one should be forced or pressured to do anything.

Animal magnetism

Our next game is foundational for developing a sense of interpersonal awareness and rapport. To begin, face your partner and define a point of contact (the back of the wrist for example), then stay connected or "sticky." At first, don't do any movement at all; just feel your body and your partner. Feel your posture and the integration of upper and lower body; feel their posture and the overall tone of their physical presence. Maybe add a little bit of strength by pushing your arm toward your partner, but just a whisper. Take your time and feel for nuance and subtlety. (You can also be "sticky" at the shoulder or the hip, side-to-side.)

Now take a breath and begin some easy, subtle movement in any direction. No matter where your partner moves, stay sticky at the point of contact. The idea is not to move in some particular way, but to feel. Slow down and sense. What is my partner saying with her body? This is the physical experience of attention and rapport. The concept is perfectly simple, but somatically sophisticated.

To make things more interesting, you can designate one person as "coach," the other as "athlete." Once sticky contact is established, the coach moves as desired, leading the athlete through a series of fluid movements. Then switch: the coach becomes the athlete and so on. Be sure to maintain eye contact. Also, be sure to switch partners frequently, as everyone has their own physical disposition and there's something to be learned from everyone.

In the advanced variation, set up facing your partner, with contact at the outside of the wrist as before. Be sticky and strong. Once you're powerfully connected, the coach advances with a shuffle step, as the athlete retreats, also with a shuffle step. The coach gives as much intensity as the athlete can handle; the idea is not to overwhelm the athlete, but to provide a powerfully integrating challenge. This is not a competition; it's a training exercise. When

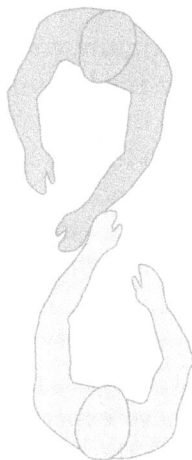

you reach the far side of the room or training area, maintain contact, but reverse roles and repeat. Try it with a variety of partners.

Animal magnetism is a fun game and is valuable on its own merits, but what's really important is the metaphor of continuity, connection, sensitivity, and what we might call physical listening. When our partners are paying attention and the rapport is strong, we feel safe; this is an ideal situation for any hypersocial primate.

But notice how it feels when someone abruptly breaks rapport, either by withdrawing (ghosting) or by moving in a way that's random, unpredictable, or jerky. It just feels wrong. You might even experience a wave of anxiety when your partner violates the physical agreement that you've established. This is the larger benefit to the practice; once you've experienced physical rapport with your partner, keep the feeling alive as you go through your day. Your partner is a model for the world at large.

Judo heckle

Our next game is more physically robust and touch-intensive, and it's great for people of all ages and fitness levels. The instructions are simple:

> "Face your partner and hold their shoulders with soft hands. You have two jobs. First, you've got to keep your partner safe. If it feels like they're about to fall over, guide them back into balance and stability. Second, it's also your responsibility to heckle your partner, mostly at the shoulder or upper arm."

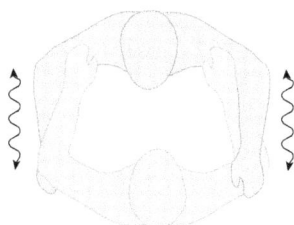

When it's clear that people understand the instructions, have them stand on one foot and begin. Instantly, things will get hilarious and people will be laughing out loud. This is a new challenge and it's wonderful in the way it allows us to take care of one another while also giving them some instability to work with. And because it challenges our physical stability, it's also fantastic for developing sensation and proprioception throughout the legs, hips, knees, and ankles.

Naturally, some people will go wild with this one and the intensity will ramp up fast. This is good fun, but it's also important to go the other way, toward slow and subtle variations. Model this for your students and coach them into sensitivity. "Fast and strong is good, but slow and smooth is good too…Make your heckles light and feel what your partner is giving you."

The beauty of the judo heckle is that it makes good use of both verbal and nonverbal communication. Coach your people to say what they need out loud. "If you want more or less intensity from your partner, say so." And be sure to have your people switch partners frequently; everyone's different in the way they move. And in this sense, everyone's a teacher, everyone's a coach.

Sidewalk dilemma

Our next exercise forces us to read the posture and motion of our partners in face-to-face encounters. This "sidewalk dilemma" is a familiar challenge for anyone who's walked down a city street. Coach your people with these instructions:

> "There's a person coming toward you and you're
> not sure of their intended path. Pay close
> attention to their posture and movement, read
> their intent and make a decision to pass left or
> right. You can pass with your bodies front-to-
> front, back-to-front, or back-to-back. The details
> don't matter as long as you do it gracefully and
> without a collision."

Next, model the encounter. Choose someone on the other side of the room or field, and walk toward them at an easy pace. Just like on a real sidewalk, you'll make a decision at some point, all based on what your body is sensing in your partner. Slide on by, take a few steps, turn around, and repeat the process.

It's easy, but things start to get really interesting when we relax and settle into the process. As people get comfortable with the challenge and develop a sense of rapport, have them increase the intensity. Shorten the distance and increase the speed as desired, but continue to focus on smooth, graceful movement.

Don't be satisfied with one or two reps on this one. Switch partners frequently and keep studying the ways that people move. There may be some minor collisions and stumbles along the way, but even then, keep the focus on fluidity and equipoise.

If you'd like to increase the challenge further, the next step is to come toward your partner with a vertical arm movement that mimics a sword strike. Slow and predictable, move your arm straight down in the sagittal plane, directly at your partner's forehead and center line.

This is more intense and intimidating, but the challenge is precisely the same as before; pass your partner left or right, sliding gracefully out of the path of the "sword." Start with plenty of distance and a predictable approach, then narrow the gap and increase the intensity. This game makes for a perfect equipoise challenge: breathe, stay calm, and slide diagonally into your partner's space, just past the arc of the sword.

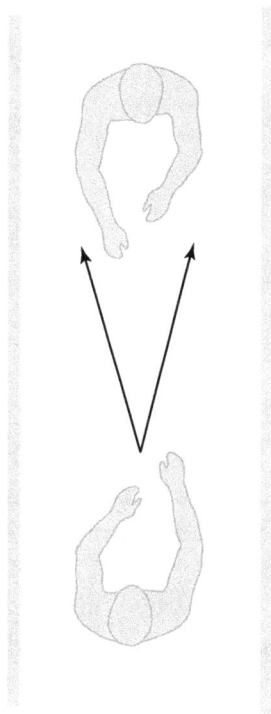

Target touch

The next game presents a solid challenge to our balance, proprioception, and stability, especially as we move in the transverse plane. And even better, it adds to our sense of rapport with one another.

Have your people pair off and designate one person as the coach, the other as the athlete. The coach's job is to hold up two hands as targets. The athlete's job is to perform cross-body touches to the targets, standing on one foot. (Or, a two-footed stance for beginners.)

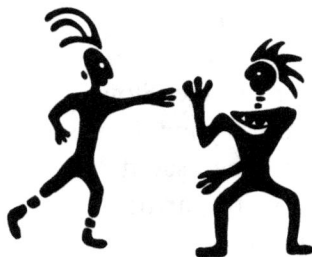

In the beginning, the coach keeps his targets close together, at shoulder height and in easy reach. At this point, the athlete typically has no problem with the challenge; the diagonal movements are modest and easy to control. But as rapport develops, the coach slowly increases the demand by widening the targets or offsetting them with one higher and one lower. This is where things begin to get really interesting and the athlete will begin to struggle.

As the master coach, you may be satisfied with this level of challenge. But if your people are doing well, you can increase the demand by asking your coaches to slowly back up. Now the challenge escalates radically; not only do your athletes have to manage the diagonal, cross-body movement, they'll also have to hop to close the distance.

This is a valuable and robust game, but there's a bit of a complication; people will get excited and they'll start moving fast. In itself, a quick pace is not a problem, but to really build balance and proprioception, the superior challenge is to go slow. Coach it this way: "Stand on one foot, feel your stability, then reach for the target with smooth, contained precision. Resist the urge to speed up. Breathe, feel, move." Do a few sets at this pace, then let people pick up the pace as desired.

Gorilla circle

Our next game is a fantastic test of position, balance, stability and physical ingenuity; plus, it's incredibly fun. Begin by outlining a circle on your floor or field, roughly six to eight feet in diameter. Draw it with chalk or something similar. (As you'll see, there's no need for precision here. You can even scratch a circle in the dirt.)

Next, get two people in the circle with these instructions:

> "OK, hands behind your back. You can contact your partner at the hip or shoulder. You can push, yield, or turn as desired. But whatever you do, stay inside the circle. Winner stays in and has a go with the next partner."

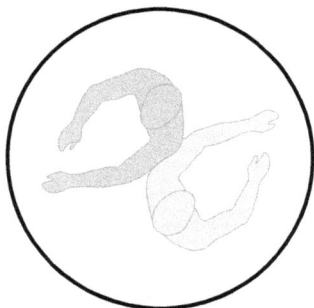

Clearly, this is a competitive contest, but there's a twist. Raw strength isn't going to win. Instead, players need to move and above all, be sensitive to the position and physical disposition of their partners. It's a classic example of maneuver in combat; intelligent yielding can sometimes defeat a more aggressive opponent. In the language of Taoism, "the weak gains victory over the strong."

Naturally, people will get excited and the enthusiasm will build fast. This is all good fun, but you'll also want to step in and dampen down the pace on occasion: "Slow it down, breathe, and take your time. Feel your posture and position. Use a gentle nudge with your hip and see how it goes." This will build sensitivity and physical intelligence.

PARTNER RESIST

Next up is partner-resist, a sophisticated relational encounter that builds rapport, strength, and stability. In conventional strength training, we use dumbbells or medicine balls to build muscular strength, but in this example we use live human bodies to give us what we need.

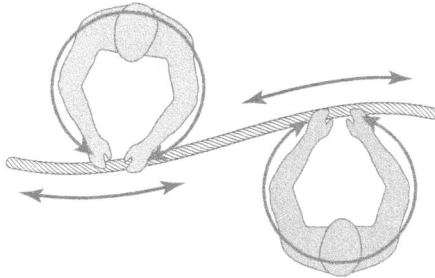

The possibilities here are endless, but in essence, you'll build on a simple movement, inviting partners to slow one another down as they try to complete the movement. Sometimes described as a "cooperative contest," this method asks participants to be both strong and yielding in motion. Technically speaking, these encounters challenge us to alternate between concentric and eccentric movements–being strong as muscles shorten *and* when they lengthen. This method is holistic, complex and physically demanding.

To get the idea, imagine a conventional "arm wrestling" contest. In the familiar, competitive model, the objective is simply to win by being as strong as possible. It's purely a zero-sum game. But in partner-resist, participants are instructed to slow one another down and make them work to complete the movement. The idea is not to defeat your opponent, but to give them a good training experience.

Almost any movement can be a candidate for partner-resist. For example, simple lateral steps are a good place to begin. Set up with your partner, shoulder-to-shoulder and hip-to-hip, facing the same direction. The athlete starts stepping sideways while the coach slows him down with smooth, even resistance. When you cross the room or the field, switch roles. Athlete becomes coach, and so on.

The beauty of this partner-resist model is that it removes competition from the process and puts the focus on sensation. Victory and defeat are no longer an issue. Instead, the focus is on relationship and physical intelligence. Partner-resist training probably builds some measure of raw strength, but more important, it builds sensitivity, adaptability, and rapport. It teaches participants to feel one another in motion and to listen to what other bodies are saying.

Even better, partner-resist encourages social give-and-take. Participants are encouraged to voice what they're looking for and to tell one another what they need. For example: "give me a little more," "slow it down," or "that's too much." This builds a sense of safety and trust.

When working with partner-resist movements, you

might assume that it's essential to have partners who are evenly matched in size and strength but, this is usually unnecessary. Since competition is no longer relevant, people of various sizes and weights can train with one another, and athletic people can train with beginners. Even with a mismatch, learning is still taking place. Every human body is different and we can all learn something new from a body in motion.

MEDITATION

> When the ocean is searching for you, don't walk to
> the language-river. Listen to the ocean, and bring
> your talky business to an end.

—Rumi

The next foundational element in our experiential design is meditation and closely related practices such as breath and somatic work. This is easy to incorporate into your practice and will give your students, athletes, or offspring some powerful mind-body benefits. In fact, meditation is an essential antidote to our modern, alien lifestyle, and makes a perfect complement to other forms of training, whether they be athletics, classroom education, or health care. It also contributes to our equipoise and equanimity in action.

In the popular narrative, meditation advocates are quick to emphasize the health and performance benefits that come with the practice. In fact, meditation does calm the body, easing us into a healing, parasympathetic state with reduced blood pressure, lower stress hormones, and all the rest. But an even more important benefit is psychological and spiritual. Fundamentally, meditation gives us experiential proof of our ability to live with ourselves, to coexist with whatever turmoil we might be experiencing. Once we learn that we can sit still with our stress, grief, confusion, and angst, these things lose some of their power to tyrannize us.

The good news is that anyone can lead the practice. If

you can say "Let's gather 'round and sit quietly for a few minutes," you're qualified. The very act of including meditation in your program will have a powerful normalizing effect for your students, clients, children, and athletes.

That said, there are some understandings that will make you a better teacher or coach. In the first place, it's essential that we keep things as simple as possible. In some settings, meditation is presented as a path to some kind of altered, exceptional state of consciousness, and while this might sometimes be the case, it also makes sense to frame it in the inverse. That is, meditation is a way to access our *normal* state of consciousness, our natural, primal state of mind and body. It's a return to our most human way of being in the world, a state before modernity, before language, before the noise, multitasking, stress, and trauma of today's world. In other words, we're not reaching for something special, we're simply letting go of all the things that get in our way.

In practice, simple is the way. Sit your people down and invite them to get comfortable and relax. In all probability, they've been hammered all day and most of their lives by people telling them to "try harder" and to be more productive. But now, you're giving them permission to "try softer." This is a time to relinquish effort. Pay attention to your breath, of course, but let the experience come to you. Soften your resistance and your striving. Be gentle. Don't try to change anything.

The fascinating thing about this practice is that our meditation sessions come to resemble the familiar progression of athletic or musical skill development that spans months and years. In the beginning, our minds are active, working hard to do whatever it is we're trying to do. We concentrate and focus on our moves, our posture, and our breath. But little by little, we let go of the effort and trust the body to do what needs to be done. We get out of the way and allow ourselves to experience *wu wei* and effortlessness.

It all makes perfect sense. Your body has a million years of evolutionary history and fundamentally, it knows what it's doing. The images, thoughts, and sensations that come to mind in meditation are nothing more than the body metabolizing its experience; this is what the body does and it's nothing to be concerned about. In a very real sense, your body can do no wrong. Just trust your it to do what it needs to do. You don't need to control it, manage it, judge it, or fight back against it. Your body is doing the best it can under the circumstances, so let it be.

SOMATIC AND BREATHWORK PRACTICES

Closely related to meditation are the various breathwork and somatic practices that you might want to include in your experiential design. All of these practices share a common objective: working with the body to ease stress, build awareness, and help people transition into a more relaxed, rest-and-digest state of being.

Breath is paramount in these efforts and in fact, when it comes to describing the power of the breath for the human animal, it's almost impossible to overstate how influential it can be. Not only does it move our vital oxygen, prana, and life force, it also guides our state of mind and spirit. Breath lies at the center, not just of the body, but our entire lived experience.

The action starts with the vagus nerve and the diaphragm, the incredible, dome-shaped muscle that lies between our abdominal and thoracic cavities. When we inhale, the muscle flattens out, massaging and gently compressing our abdominal organs. On exhalation, the diaphragm relaxes and returns to its dome-like shape. It's a beautiful, elegant, even awe-inspiring system.

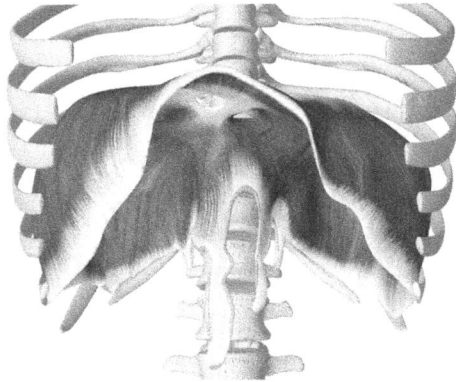

Sadly, modern life tends to compromise our natural, health-positive breath patterns. Under assault by chronic stress, our breath becomes shallow, weak, and ineffective. The diaphragm fails to work through its full range, and everything in our body and mind suffers as a result.

The cures are various but well within our capability. In fact, the animal body tends to do the right thing naturally, without special training. Before or after stressful events, the body is usually smart enough to take a big breath, followed by a long, slow exhale, and in the process, we feel a bit better. Given enough time and opportunity, the human animal will generally take care of itself, but occasionally we need extra help and sometimes, we're so deep in stress that we need reminders of what normal breath actually feels like.

With this in mind, you might want to include some

remedial breath practices in your programs. The details aren't particularly important, and it's surely the case that almost all breathwork is valuable. For example, you might do a session that emphasizes long, slow exhales; this has been shown to activate the rest-and-digest, or feed-breed response. Or, you might include "box breathing," with equal time (three or four seconds, as desired) spent inhaling, holding, exhaling, and holding. There's also a practice called "cyclic sighing" that involve inhaling slowly and then inhaling a bit more to fully fill the lungs before slowly exhaling. No matter which practice you choose, it's all good work.

Progressive relaxation

Closely related to breathwork are the various stress-relieving practices of progressive relaxation. The point here is to bring awareness to the body and to turn on the parasympathetic branch of the autonomic nervous system, the branch devoted to tissue healing and repair, what neurobiologist Robert Sapolsky calls "the long-term rebuilding projects."

A typical session is built on a set of simple mind-body prompts and suggestions. Gather your people together, seated or lying down. Once they're settled, begin the prompts, with lots of emphasis on the breath.

There's no set way to do this, but whatever you choose to do, take plenty of time in your delivery:

Once you're comfortable, start with some easy breaths...

Inhale with your whole body. Expand, relax

completely....

Inhale...exhale and let all the tension drain from your body....

Let the floor do all the work of supporting you....

Inhale....exhale and let every cell in your body relax....

Feel your hands...heavy and warm...heavy and warm....

And so on. Don't be afraid to repeat any instruction. Take your time and use a voice that's quiet and comforting.

Or, you can go system by system, improvising as desired:

Feel all the bones in your body. Feel their weight, their mass. Exhale... let them relax....

Take a breath.... feel the long bones in your legs...let them relax....

Take a breath.... exhale and let your pelvis relax....

Inhale.... exhale....and let your spine relax...

And so on, all the way up the body to the skull...

Or, you can emphasize the cardiovascular system:

Take a breath...exhale and allow the chambers of your heart to relax...

Inhale... exhale... feel all the blood vessels in your body and let them relax...

Inhale... exhale and let all the capillaries in your body relax...

Or, you can emphasize the nervous system:

Inhale...relax... feel your nervous system....your spinal cord, and all the nerves that span your body...

Next, address the muscles, one region at a time...

Inhale... relax and feel all your muscles and allow them to relax....

Inhale and relax... feel your quads and let them relax completely....

Feel your hamstrings....

Feel the muscles of your neck, your head, your jaw....

And so on....

Inhale and relax completely... feel all the connective tissue in your body and allow it to relax....

Feel the organs in your abdomen and allow them to relax....

And so on...

In this process, you might also choose to emphasize the interior space of various body parts, imagining vast caverns that become even bigger with each inhalation:

Inhale and relax... feel the space inside your right leg....

Take a deep breath and feel the space inside your abdomen....

Feel the space inside your chest....an enormous chamber that gets even bigger with each inhalation...

And so on, all the way through the body.

Or, you might also do a series of contract-relax efforts, each one directed at a specific body part or segment. For example:

Once you're relaxed and comfortable, direct your attention to your right foot...

Gently contract your toes...hold the contraction for a moment and then relax... let all the tension drain from your foot....

Take a deep breath, relax again, and direct your attention to your left foot... gently contract and then relax...

Ride the relaxation with your whole body...

And so on, all the way up the body, segment by segment, muscle by muscle. This will help people become more aware of any tension that they're holding and help them feel the wave of relaxation that comes with each release.

Once you've gotten your people fully relaxed, another fascinating practice is to invite them to extend their experience of relaxation to areas outside their skin. This is a particularly powerful practice that can go a long way to easing us out of chronic stress.

Start with any kind of relaxation, with whatever prompts you like. Focus on the breath as usual and take plenty of time to sink into a state of whole-body relaxation. Take plenty of time in this phase.

When your people are fully immersed in relaxation, invite them to gradually extend their sense of relaxation outward, beginning with the air just outside their bodies:

> *Inhale... exhale.... now relax the air just around your skin... feel it soften...*

Give this some time, then continue outward, taking plenty of time to address and relax the concentric spheres that surround the body...

> *Inhale... exhale... relax the room you're sitting in...*

> *Inhale... exhale... relax your neighborhood and your local habitat*

> *Inhale... exhale... relax the people and the conflict in your life...*

> *Inhale...exhale... relax the entire world...*

Keep going as far as you like, all the way to the large-scale spheres of humanity and the planet as a whole. You can even extend your relaxation all the way to the stars of the night sky, the galaxies, and the cosmos as a whole. It might sound outlandish, but it works. Just keep relaxing all of it, and if you get distracted simply return to your breath.

YUTORI

No matter which breath or bodywork practice you choose, it's essential to create a comfortable tone and pace. Just as with any rest-and-digest practice, the tone should be one of safety, permission, and an abundance of time. This is where the Japanese concept of *yutori* becomes especially valuable.

Several translations are in circulation. Some call it "spaciousness," "room to breathe," or "leeway." Others have called it "the art of unhurried spaciousness," "room in your mind," and even "margin of maneuver." But no matter what we call it, this orientation is vital not just for meditation, breathwork, and progressive relaxation, but for developing our equipoise in the wider world.

Like *wu wei*, our sense of *yutori* can be strengthened with training; it's the natural consequence of neuroplasticity and experience in our chosen art forms. The progression is simple: For beginners, time seems to be in short supply and everything feels like a rush. There are myriad patterns, tasks, sensations, and movements to be absorbed and mastered, so we hurry, trying our best to grasp the skills in question.

But over time, we become increasingly familiar with the challenge; our skills increase, but so too does our sense of time available, our *yutori*. Urgency fades away as a sense of temporal affluence and abundance unfolds. There's space in between the notes now; we know what's coming and we can relax in that knowledge.

As coaches, teachers, parents, and leaders, we cultivate *yutori* by directing the attention of our students and athletes. Talk about pace and the journey from urgency to abundance. "Yes, you're overwhelmed now, but in a few weeks or months it's going to feel different. You're going to find more space in between the challenges. You're going to find time to breathe, and the more relaxed you feel, the better your performance is going to be."

ゆとり

Likewise, we develop a sense of *yutori* in our students and athletes by modeling it and living it. Naturally, we're excited about our teaching and coaching, and we want to deliver everything we can for our people and in the beginning, we too are driven by our personal sense of urgency. Time is short, we believe, so we double down on our efforts and try to squeeze ever more content and experience into the available time.

But the hurry disease almost always fails. Urgency feeds on itself in a positive feedback cycle of rushing, error, half-measures, insensitivity, and desperate lurching for completion. Even worse, it's infectious; when coaches, teachers, and parents rush from one task to another, students, athletes, and children are sure to be swept up in the process. And no one likes to be around jumpy, frenetic people; it's just too stressful.

But of course it all goes the other way. When coaches and teachers slow down and pay attention to process, even in the face of external demands, students and athletes are likely to get the message, even unconsciously. In other words, equipoise and a relaxed mind-body start at the top. Create some "unhurried spaciousness" in your practice and your *yutori* will be contagious. Relaxation will become your superpower.

PRESENTATION

The next common element in experiential design involves the presentations that you'll give to your assembled clients, students, or athletes. This can be a powerful practice but naturally, it's also where many of us fall apart. Public speaking is stressful for most of us, and we're quick to look for an escape, or at least some measure of protection against the exposure.

This is also why so many spoken presentations are nearly unendurable. Afraid to say what we really mean, we fall back on soft language, equivocation, defensive statements, passive voice, and garbled messaging. It's no wonder that so many listeners reach for their phones.

To give a good presentation, you've got to overcome these doubts. Seize the opportunity and say what you mean with clarity and passion. Concentrate on your content and message and, in particular, why you think it's important. To put it another way, concentrate on being you. What do *you* really care about? What's truly meaningful to you? Trying to adopt the tone, content, or delivery of someone else is doomed to failure. As they say in the presentation game, "Be yourself. Everyone else is already taken."

This is also a good time to think about your role, your identity, and your objectives. It's sometimes said that there are really only two kinds of presenters: one says—either explicitly or implicitly—"I really want you to know this material," while the other says, "I really want you to know *that* I know this material." The first presenter is offering a sincere gift to the audience; the second is simply showing off. Obviously, some display of competence and mastery will add to your credibility, but ultimately, your presentation needs to be about the needs of your people, not you.

Next comes your preparation and a simple rule of thumb: An effective presentation is built on a foundation of reason and an orderly sequence. Once you've got this in place, you're free to expound with emotion, color, and passion. The writer Lyman Beecher put it this way: "Eloquence is logic on fire." In other words, use an outline and review your ideas to be sure that they make sense in sequence. Does the first idea lead to the next? Is there some kind of continuity? Are the transitions smooth or abrupt? Once you get the logic right, you can relax, adding examples, stories, and texture as desired. The tighter your reasoning, the more passionate you can be.

Sadly, this is where many of us go astray. If you've been trained at the university level, personal expression might feel alien and in fact, you might have been discouraged from presenting much of anything besides raw, objective data. And, as linguist George Lakoff points out, many of us are trained to believe that facts are persuasive on their own; if we're accurate and truthful in our statements, the audience will be convinced. We may even come to look down on the idea of selling ideas through metaphor or emotion. Lakoff calls this "the enlightenment fallacy."

Consultants in the world of public speaking make a similar observation, as marine biologist-turned filmmaker Randy Olson points out in *Don't Be Such a Scientist: Talking Substance in an Age of Style.* As Olson sees it, scientists are trained to use a particular style of language with a particular mission: the transmission and presentation of methods, findings, and data. Facts are supposed to speak for themselves, but most people outside the university community don't listen this way. In fact, humans are moved first and foremost by feeling and stories.

All of which suggests that if we're going to be effective, we need to avoid the disembodied, Cartesian speaking style that puts data front and center. These presentations do serve a specialized purpose but are death to public persuasion. Graphs, charts, and mathematical equations only work for people trained in that domain; for everyone else, they feel like punishment.

Above all, tell a story. Following the proven method of Hollywood screenwriters, start with some kind of trouble, an inciting incident that somehow disrupts the flow of routine life. There's a crime, a mystery, an illness, a trauma, a surprise, something that's broken, something that just doesn't add up. Your job as a presenter is to describe this predicament, then weave your story from there. You've got your audience's attention now, and you're ready to make your case. Take your people on a journey of exploration or explanation and try to bring some illumination back to the original predicament.

This is also a good time to think about the duration of your talk. In the world of comedy, a truism holds that "The longer the fuse, the bigger the bang must be." In other words, if the setup for your story, punch line, or explanatory climax takes a long time, you'd better be coming across with something truly exciting. For listeners, there's nothing worse than having to endure a long, laborious setup, only to be ghosted by a nonevent at the end. This is particularly true in an age of diminishing attention spans; as soon as you start taking side trips or droning on about detail, people are going to check out.

All of which brings up the issue of practice and the baffling, widespread belief that preparation and practice for public speaking is somehow unnecessary—just show up with your slide deck and you're good to go. But public speaking is no different than any other art or discipline; quality reps are the name of the game. Think of it like an athletic event; you've got to put in the time, in advance, over and over again until you get it right. This means actually speaking the words and listening to the result. Read your script out loud and give your presentation to your dog or the trees in the park. Do it again and again, over-preparing so you won't be flustered when faced with the inevitable surprises.

THE CURSE OF KNOWLEDGE

Having taken a good look at the vital elements of a classic or prototypical experiential design, there's one more issue that demands our attention, and that's the paradoxical nature of mastery and teaching itself. You've spent years honing your skills and put in thousands of hours of practice. You've integrated the experience into your body and, in the process, you might have even achieved an occasional sense of *wu wei* and effortless action. The skills and knowledge that you've worked so hard to attain now seem completely obvious and self-evident. To you, that is.

The problem is that it's one thing to know your stuff and it's something else entirely to coach or teach others what you know. What's obvious to you may seem not just difficult but maybe even impossible to beginners. This is what psychologist Steven Pinker has called the curse of knowledge. It's "the difficulty in imagining what it's like for someone else not to know something that you know."

Take the alphabet for example. You've been working with it for decades and you rarely if ever stop to question it in any way. You're completely fluent, and the process seems entirely self-evident. Any fool can see how it works, and you're likely to get frustrated with anyone who fails to grasp it instantly. The same goes for the fundamentals in any art: musical chords and scales, athletic movements, technical skills, and so on. Our experience gives us a sense of intimate, tissue-level familiarity with the art, but to the beginner, it may well seem mysterious, baffling, and even completely out of reach.

All of which makes coaching and teaching intrinsically problematic and even frustrating. We wonder how beginners can be so slow, so obtuse, so dull. Why can't they see what is so clearly evident? This also explains why master performers aren't necessarily good teachers or coaches, and that some are simply horrible. They've fully integrated their skills into their bodies and they can't understand how anyone could fail to see the obvious. In some cases, they can't even remember what it was like to not know the material or the movements. As a result, they have little patience for anyone who can't see what they see or feel what they feel.

In turn, this suggests an entirely new orientation for coaching and teaching. Yes, of course, we need some competence with the skills involved and it's important that we've made the journey ourselves. But teaching demands a certain kind of memory and an appreciation for the beginner's struggle. In other words, teachers and coaches need to forget what's obvious. They need to forget the skills that they've worked so hard to attain and ignore the fact that it now feels so effortless.

Instead, the challenge is to remember and appreciate the awkwardness, the confusion, and the struggles that go with being a beginner. In turn, this becomes a kind of competence and skill in itself. Fundamentally, it's an act of imagination, compassion, and above all, patience. It also forces us to re-engineer the learning sequences and fundamentals that lead the novice into skill. What are the fundamentals anyway? What are the most vital first steps? What are the most important reps for the young person or novice? How do we establish the neurological watercourse that will lead students and athletes to skill and mastery?

In other words, the career arc of the teacher and coach has two distinct phases. The first is simple skill development and mastery, but the second is a return to the basics of the learning process. In other words, it's not enough to be skilled; you've got to remember and honor your original awkwardness and incompetence. Remember how hard it was to grasp the fundamentals. Now imagine someone who's struggling and step into their shoes. What will it take to get them on the path to *wu wei*?

CHAPTER 8

THE LONG GAME

Hope is not the conviction that something will turn out well, but the certainty that something is worth doing no matter how it turns out.

—Václav Havel

Czech dissident and statesman

So you've done the work. You've crafted your experiential design and set the process in motion. You've focused on your objectives and you're intent on developing highly functional, competent, and creative human animals. Maybe you're planning on doing basic one-hour classes or more ambitious multi-day workshops. Or maybe you're just incorporating some new understandings into what you're already doing.

In any case, there are going to be times when things come together and it's going to feel like magic. Your planning and organization will click into place and you'll feel a powerful sense of *wu wei* and effortless action. Your people will be engaged and energized; your teaching will spark their curiosity and feed their hunger. They'll be delighted with the rapport they build with one another, and the end result will be transformative and inspiring. This is what you live for.

But like Mama said, there are going to be days when things go sideways. Surprises are everywhere. Your facility might be unavailable at the last minute, your technology will develop glitches, or your people will come to you with a raft of concerns that simply must be addressed. Some of your efforts will strike home, but other parts of your message will dissolve into noise, confusion, or worse. It's going to be a mixed bag.

No matter your background or best intentions, you're going to get some things wrong along the way. You'll mess up on the planning, people will show up late, there won't be enough food, you'll get side-tracked in your presentation, and your computer will crash at the worst possible moment.

And naturally, all of this will take a toll on your equanimity. Your attention will fragment and your focus will be compromised. You might even have to revise your plan midstream to compensate for unforeseen events. And of course, you'll almost certainly blame yourself for everything that goes wrong.

GOOD WORK

At times like these, it's essential to remember that your work is both valuable and honorable. You may never be recognized for what you do, and some will even scoff that you've chosen such an unprofitable, humanitarian path. Incredibly, your passionate interest in the welfare of the human animal might even make you feel like an outlier. Your work, precious and important as it is, may well be passed over by the latest sensation, the latest gizmo, or the latest celebrity. Oddly and tragically, your work with might even be dismissed as just another low-profit, non-profit, feel-good enterprise, scarcely worthy of consideration. And when you tell people what you're up to, they'll ask the inevitable: "Do you want fries with that?"

But remember, this assessment is not about you; it's about society. Your status, or rather lack of status, is a reflection of a perverse value system that puts profit above both planet and people. So don't forget: Teaching is one of the most honorable practices that human beings have ever engaged in, and you're part of that lineage. Even in an age when human knowledge lives in server farms and is available at the touch of button, humans will always need one another in face-to-face encounters. In other words, your work is vital, honorable, and more than ever, essential.

PANORAMA

Your journey into experiential design, teaching, and leadership may not play out in the way you imagine. You might suppose that with experience you'll gain a sense of confidence and become progressively smarter and more effective in everything you do. You'll gain a firmer grasp of your objectives, your content, and your methods, and in this sense at least, you'll succeed. You might even gain a sense of equipoise and *wu wei*.

But oddly, the process often seems to go the other way entirely. As we gain experience, we find ourselves becoming increasingly aware of our limitations and our deficiencies. There's so much to be taught and so much to be said, and there's never enough time to do it all. Along the way, we're astonished to find ourselves floundering and feeling unsure of our footing. At times like this, we might well come to appreciate the view of historian and philosopher

Will Durant, who quipped, "Education is the progressive discovery of our own ignorance."

Durant was surely right, but we also can reframe his observation to say that "Education is the progressive discovery of the vastness of our enterprise." In other words, our new orientation comes not from our *lack* of understanding but from a growing appreciation for depth and breadth of our endeavor, the realization that the scope of our discipline is far bigger than we'd first imagined. It's not the case that we're becoming increasingly inept or incompetent, but rather that the horizon of our imagination is growing with each passing season. We see more complexity, more nuance, more interdependence and, in the process, the world becomes a bigger, richer, and more fascinating place.

The mountain climb is the perfect metaphor. We struggle and sweat to go higher, and every now and then we turn around to admire the view. With each step, the panorama gets more expansive, the world becomes more magnificent. But we don't conquer the mountain at all; in fact, just the reverse. The mountain conquers our ego and our sense of importance. By the time we reach the summit, the world appears enormous, just as we become vividly aware of our personal insignificance. It's not so much that we feel ignorant but rather that we become part of something greater. As the Norwegian philosopher Arne Næss put it, "The smaller we come to feel ourselves compared to the mountain, the nearer we come to participating in its greatness."

ELDERSHIP

As you gain experience in your work and your chosen profession, you'll probably define yourself with familiar labels like "coach," "therapist," or "teacher," but you'll also be growing into a leadership role and perhaps, something of a tribal elder. You've spent years in study and engagement, learned valuable lessons, and you're ready to share them with your people—people who might even come to respect your contribution to their welfare and the future.

But then again, maybe not. As it stands, there's something seriously amiss with our modern narrative about seniority, aging, and respect. Everyone knows the prevailing story that circulates through our culture and our collective unconscious: Aging is one long, depressing decline into degeneration, illness, and loneliness. Certain events are said to be inevitable: decreased physical and cognitive function, massive medical bills, neurological meltdown, and perhaps worst of all, social and cultural irrelevance. In short, getting older is a slow motion train wreck to be avoided by any means necessary.

But the personal, social, and cultural consequences of this narrative are catastrophic. Not only does it make us increasingly miserable and fearful as time goes by, it also drives the widespread practice of ageism. We don't really respect our seniors in the modern world and, more likely, we view them as nothing more than a drag on society and the economy. In our eyes, human value peaks in young adulthood, then decreases sharply over time.

But in the context of human history, this kind of narrative is profoundly deviant. In a historically normal, Paleo world, tribal survival was highly dependent on the experience, knowledge, and wisdom of the elders. The old ones had participated in many hunts and observed the waxing and waning of animal life over the course of decades; they'd seen the tribe suffer and flourish through good times and bad. In this context, their words and judgment carried enormous weight. As keepers of vital knowledge, they were the most valuable and respected members of the community. In the Paleolithic world, human value increased over time. This is why Native Americans still say, "When an elder dies, a library burns."

In the Old Way, the elders were fully aware of their role and their responsibility. Experience in wild outdoor environments made it clear: The primary duty of the elder was to act on behalf of the tribe, to share their knowledge, to give away their insights so the tribe could live another day, perhaps another year. There would have been no thought of retirement, no notion of self-pampering, or hoarding of knowledge as a commodity to be bought and sold. For the Paleolithic senior citizen, the primal directive was simple: Give away your wisdom so the tribe can live.

In essence, the tribal elder is the ultimate servant leader. As she looks out at the immensity of the world outside of camp, she feels the exposure and the vulnerability. She knows how hard it is just to stay alive. She worries about the state of her people and what it will take to keep them whole. Has she done all she can to help them navigate the world? Do the young hunters know all they need to know about the ways of the animals, the weather, and the threats from neighboring tribes? What else must she teach before she goes?

As a servant leader, the tribal elder understands her life and health in a unique way, one that will come as a surprise to modern ears. In today's culture, we're bombarded with messages, products, and services designed to keep us forever young. Heeding this call, we do everything possible to maximize our individual welfare. We focus on ourselves, our training, and our bodies. We try to hoard our health and keep it intact as long as possible.

But for the tribal elder, the purpose of health is not to hoard it but to give it away. Give it away to the tribe and loved ones, so they can carry on. Give it away so that your people might thrive. Of course your body will start to decay. Of course you will die. But by giving our health to the world, we fulfill our role and her purpose. What else is health for, if not to spend it on the people and causes that need it?

This is why, as an aspiring tribal elder, it's perfectly appropriate to offer life lessons to your students, clients, and athletes. Typically, these are short, pithy conversations about how to live, often given at the end of a movement or meditation session. It's common practice in the world of yoga, some athletic training, and is very much a part of the martial art tradition. Your students and athletes have done some vigorous movement or meditation, their bodies are fluid and relaxed, and they're likely to be receptive to some words of wisdom. In fact, people crave this kind of guidance, especially at this moment in history.

You may not think of yourself as a particularly wise leader, and you might be reluctant to offer life lessons at all; in all probability, you're trying to figure things out for yourself. But this is precisely the reason to speak up. People are looking to you for some kind of direction and they want to hear what you have to say. And if you don't feel that you have answers, you can at least offer questions. Even framing a life issue in a particular way, without offering solutions, can be powerful. Don't miss this opportunity. For some of your clients, students, and athletes, this may ultimately prove to be the most influential and impactful part of the entire experience, so you've got to be brave and make the effort.

Of course, being a tribal elder—even an aspiring tribal elder—is no easy path. The problem is that you're probably not going to be rewarded for your efforts, not in a conventional sense, and almost certainly not in your lifetime. The events you set in motion today might take a long time to play out, and successful outcomes might not materialize for years or decades.

In other words, your work is highly speculative and in rational, economic terms, somewhat absurd. What kind of fool would invest in an outcome she will never see or experience? But this is not rational economics; it's something deeper and more powerful. And in this domain, sacrificing for a distant, tribal good isn't folly—it's an act of sapience. Giving one's life for downstream improvement not only feeds the greater good, it also makes us happier and healthier as individuals in *this* lifetime.

If you're looking for a quick payoff, you're in the wrong line of work. Instead, take your sense of satisfaction directly from the activity itself and from the meaning that it holds. Connect with the intrinsic pleasures that come with teaching and coaching: working with people, organizing, creating curriculum, and crafting narratives. It's a tough gig, but big, audacious goals require a long view. As the American theologian Reinhold Niebuhr put it, "Nothing that is worth doing can be achieved in our lifetime."

A WHY TO LIVE

As with all truly creative endeavors, there are going to be obstacles, stressors, and hardships along the way. You're trying to do something unique, something outside the realm of convention, and not everyone is going to understand or appreciate your vision. Especially in an age of escalating stress, your people will show a strong, almost unstoppable urge to revert to familiar culture, practices, rituals, themes, and belief systems. The last thing people want is something innovative and challenging. More likely, they want to be comforted.

All of which might well leave you out in the cold, wondering how it is that your precious shoots of optimism aren't being recognized and appreciated. You've worked hard, put in the time, and taken some substantial risks, and you're right to feel challenged by it all. But action is the antidote to our despair. Step back as necessary, take all the rest you need, then redouble your efforts. Focus, over and over again, on your *ikigai*, your sense of meaning and purpose. Focus on the work and the process itself, not its reception. Are your efforts consistent with what you're trying to create? Do they align with the story you're telling about the world and your place in it?

Many of us have heard about the power of *ikigai* by way of philosopher Friedrich Nietzsche: "He who has a why to live can endure almost any how." If we've got a mission and a sense of purpose, it's a lot easier to tolerate the slings and arrows of outrageous fortune. This was also the insight of Viktor Frankl, recounted in his classic *Man's Search for Meaning*. As he suffered brutal conditions in a Nazi concentration camp, Frankl realized that prisoners who survived were those with a strong sense of meaning and purpose. It's a powerful idea, but we might also frame it in the inverse, as in "He who lacks a why to live will be derailed by every passing distraction, annoyance, and inconvenience." Or, as the Bhagavad Gita puts it, "Those who commit to nothing are distracted by everything," a truly apt description for millions in the modern world.

Likewise, it's essential to remember that stories, no matter their origin or nature, are reps. Every time we hear or tell a story, our bodies and nervous systems are literally transformed. The effects are microscopic and subtle but immensely consequential. As we've seen, the human nervous system is constantly remodeling itself as it attempts to adapt to the world around it, and stories play right into this process. Every story we tell or hear—especially those with emotional impact—produces a distinct neuroendocrine response in the body. With every telling, the brain becomes more receptive to the associated meanings and, in turn, creates the beginning of a watercourse. With each retelling or rereading, human attention becomes more likely to follow along and deepen the grooves, for better or for worse.

In this sense, repeated tellings and listenings are no different from the reps we perform with dumbbells in the gym. Listen to a story once and we might be momentarily moved, but listen to that story a hundred times and our bodies begin to change. In turn, our transformation will touch the bodies and minds of people around us and will even be passed from one generation to the next. In other words, our stories don't just carve grooves in our bodies and brains; they also carve grooves in the future.

This is why authentic stories of meaning and purpose are so vital. So choose wisely, dig deep, and repeat the process often. Consider your values and your deepest curiosities. Is there a why that will sustain you through any how? Is there a vision or a purpose that can keep you going, even in times of chaos, confusion, or stress? Is there a story that will help sustain your equanimity and equipoise in the face of ambiguity and uncertainty?

Find that purpose and make it your own. Live life on your terms and follow your curiosities. Don't be content with plastic stories and synthetic narratives that tell you what to value and how to live. Even in the face of stress and adversity, it's better to fail in your chosen art then to succeed with an artificial sense of meaning and purpose. As Fyodor Dostoyevsky put it, "To go wrong in one's own way is better than to go right in someone else's."

THE TEACHING IS YOU

> The world is changed by your example, not by your opinion.
>
> Paulo Coelho, novelist

As we get deeper into our teaching and coaching journey, we gain expertise with our content, our programs, and our presentations. We refine our work and we're proud of the result. Along the way, we might even be tempted to think that we've gained a sense of mastery.

But in the long run, it's important to remember that the ultimate teaching is not your content, nor is it your slideshow, your team-building games, your handouts, or your exercises. Rather, the teaching is *you*. It's the way you live and the way you show up that makes the difference in people's lives. In other words, you're not just someone who designs, manages, or presents a program. *You* are the content and the curriculum.

To be sure, your students, clients, and athletes will probably be interested in your material and how it's presented, but at the end of the day, they're hypersocial animals, which is to say, their greatest curiosity is people. They want to know who you are and how you live. In this spirit, Coach John Wooden often quoted a passage by Rudyard Kipling: "No written word, no spoken plea can teach our youth what they should be; nor all the books on all the shelves—it's what the teachers are themselves."

This is particularly true at this moment in history, when chaos and uncertainty escalate with each passing day. Long-established structures are breaking down and ambiguity is everywhere. Traditional rituals and guardrails are weakening, and people are left to wonder: How are we to live in an age of ecological and social incoherence? How do my teachers and coaches manage it? Are they feeling what I'm feeling? How are they managing their anxiety about the world? Can I model my life after theirs or should I look elsewhere for guidance and inspiration?

It's a weighty responsibility, and you're bound to wonder about what you're doing and what kind of effect you're having on the world; on bad days you might even wonder if you're having any effect at all. After all, there's no real way to know what your people are going to do in the weeks, months, and years after they train with you.

But this is just how it goes when you're working with complex systems. Actions have consequences, but it's hard to track the precise course of cause and effect. In fact, butterfly effects are everywhere in our work; biospheres, social systems, and human nervous systems are similar in the way that small, seemingly insignificant actions can multiply into enormous downstream consequences.

And while we can't exercise direct control over how the future unfolds, we *can* control how we show up. If we've got the right spirit and the right sincerity, we can rest assured that there will be a positive downstream effect; we just don't know the details. In this sense, it makes sense to view our lives as an endless series of butterfly effects. If we keep showing up with sincerity, humility, and resolve, rest assured, there will be positive downstream consequences.

The ancients knew this well. For thousands of years, our elders taught that the ultimate practice is to show up in the world with the right posture, attitude, balance, and equipoise. In this practice, sincerity is everything. You'll make mistakes, but error is just error. Like drummers in the circle, we're going to miss the beat and play the wrong notes—more often than we'd like. But this is nothing to be concerned about; it's simply your nervous system reaching for skill. If you keep showing up with sincerity, you're doing it right.

Likewise, this teaching inspires a sense of humility in our practice. Even when we succeed in mastering a particular skill, we remain as short-lived humans, completely susceptible to self-deception, cognitive biases, social contagion, current events, placebo and nocebo effects, environmental influence, and the arc of history. In other words, mastery is an illusion. No matter how skillful and experienced we become, we remain vulnerable to the forces of culture, biology, and psychology. At our best and our worst, we are nothing more or less than fallible creators.

So we walk the path and we keep showing up. On good days, our engagement feels satisfying and even magical. Our people are moving steadily toward *wu wei*; they're curious, attentive, and delighted in the rapport they're developing with the process and one another. But there are going to be days when nothing goes right. Your students will disrespect you, your colleagues will ghost you, and it's going to feel like the entire world is lining up to sabotage your efforts. You're going to feel angry, depressed, alienated, and outraged. You'll even think about leaving the game entirely.

But it's all part of the process. Showing up means showing up in all conditions, no matter our reservations, or our fears. This is the spiritual practice, bringing our best game to the encounter, even when we're compromised and distracted, even when we'd much rather be doing something else. In these conditions, it's tempting to reach for some kind of escape, but courage is always the better choice. Anarchist Edward Abbey once called courage the master virtue because, as he saw it, "Without courage, all other virtues are useless." If you're stepping up with whatever you've got, you're doing the right thing.

So be tenacious and stick with the process. Take all the time you need for rest and recovery, but above all, keep showing up with all the equipoise you can muster. Along the way, remember the wisdom of coach Wooden: Practice *is* the destination. If you're giving it your best effort each day, you're in the sweet spot of teaching, coaching, leadership, and life. As Mahatma Gandhi put it, "Satisfaction lies in the effort, not in the attainment, full effort is full victory."

RECOMMENDED READING

Your path to mastery in experiential design is sure to cover lots of territory, with plenty of diversions, side trips, and occasional dead-ends. And as Heraclitus taught, "We can't step into the same river twice." Each year will bring new insights and perspectives on what it means to be a coach, teacher, parent, or leader in your field. This is what makes the journey so fascinating. Even after decades of work, you'll still be re-creating and fine-tuning your philosophy and programs to fit the needs of your people and the world at large.

Nevertheless, there are some foundational works that will help you shape your understanding and your practice. Here's a reading list to get you started:

The Aims of Education by Alfred North Whitehead

Awareness Through Movement: Easy-to-Do Health Exercises to Improve Your Posture, Vision, Imagination, and Personal Awareness by Moshe Feldenkrais

The Body Keeps the Score: Brain, Mind, and Body in the Healing of Trauma by Bessel van der Kolk

Drumming at the Edge of Magic: A Journey into the Spirit of Percussion by Mickey Hart and Jay Stevens

Effortless Mastery: Liberating the Master Musician Within by Kenny Werner

Finite and Infinite Games: A Vision of Life as Play and Possibility by James P. Carse

Flow: The Psychology of Optimal Experience by Mihaly Csikszentmihalyi

The Forgotten Power of Rhythm by Reinhard Flatischler

Free Play: Improvisation in Life and Art by Stephen Nachmanovitch

Mindset: The New Psychology of Success by Carol Dweck

The Myth of Normal: Trauma, Illness, and Healing in a Toxic Culture by Gabor Maté

The Neurobiology of We: How Relationships, the Mind, and the Brain Interact to Shape Who We Are by Daniel Siegel

The Old Way: A Story of the First People by Elizabeth Marshall Thomas

The Plastic Mind: New Science Reveals Our Extraordinary Potential to Transform Ourselves by Sharon Begley

Punished by Rewards: The Trouble with Gold Stars, Incentive Plans, A's, Praise, and Other Bribes by Alfie Kohn

Rhythms of Life: The Biological Clocks That Control the Daily Lives of Every Living Thing by Russell Foster and Leon Kreitzman

Surviving Survival: The Art and Science of Resilience by Laurence Gonzales

Tao Te Ching by Lao Tzu

Why Zebras Don't Get Ulcers: The Acclaimed Guide to Stress, Stress-Related Diseases, and Coping by Robert Sapolsky

The Wisdom of Insecurity: A Message for an Age of Anxiety by Alan Watts

The Wisdom of No Escape: and the Path of Loving Kindness by Pema Chödrön

The Book of Chuang Tzu

GRATITUDE

Writing any book is hard enough, but as anyone who writes about our ecological and humanitarian crisis knows, our words often fall on deaf ears. We make the best presentation we can, but people are reading fewer books these days and denial seems to be trending.

In the process, we're likely to feel like Cassandra, the Trojan priestess dedicated to the god Apollo, fated to utter true prophecies but never to be believed. We stand up and speak out, but in a culture that, in the words of media critic Neil Postman, is "amusing ourselves to death," we're often ignored and marginalized.

So it's easy to fall into despair and naturally, we need all the help we can get. The good news is that I've been massively supported—directly and indirectly—by a host of truly exceptional people who've helped me navigate the darkness. In particular, I'd like to extend my deepest gratitude to:

Danny McMillian

Rodney King

John Hagar

Jonathan Logan

Jennifer Rioux

Dana Lyons

Max Wilbert

Fode Sylla and the drummers of Bend, Oregon
Louie and Gerlinde Gelina
Oz Marginean and the True Athlete Project
Jill Stephenson
Amelia and Taryn DuBose
George Tsakraklides
Alessandro Pelizzon
David Kopacz
Diedre Knowlton and Barb Moro
Elizabeth Dougherty
Vern Gambetta
Pete Karabetis
Michael Campi
Corey Jung
Marisa Solis
Steve Laskevitch and Carla Fraga
James O'Keefe
Paul Landon
Stuart Brown
Derrick Jensen
Cari Taylor
Alex Gientke
Ron Kauk
The love of my life, Sue Schwantes
And finally Mojo, the alpha Labrador,
may he rest in peace.

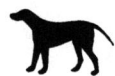